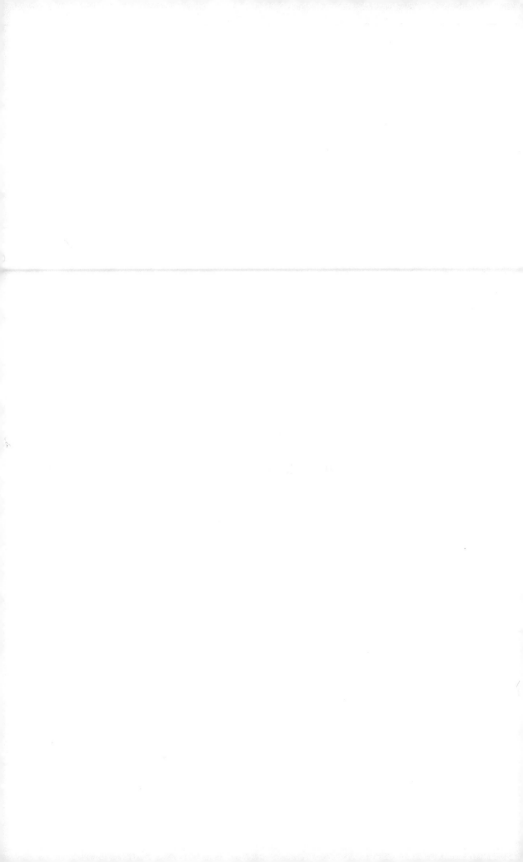

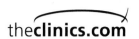

theclinics.com

DENTAL CLINICS
OF NORTH AMERICA

Dental Materials

GUEST EDITORS
Lyle D. Zardiackas, PhD, FADM,
Tracy M. Dellinger, DDS, MS, and
Mark Livingston, DDS

July 2007 • Volume 51 • Number 3

SAUNDERS

An Imprint of Elsevier, Inc.
PHILADELPHIA LONDON TORONTO MONTREAL SYDNEY TOKYO

W.B. SAUNDERS COMPANY
A Division of Elsevier Inc.

Elsevier Inc. • 1600 John F. Kennedy Boulevard • Suite 1800 • Philadelphia, Pennsylvania 19103-2899

http://www.dental.theclinics.com

DENTAL CLINICS OF NORTH AMERICA	**Volume 51, Number 3**
July 2007	**ISSN 0011-8532**
Editor: John Vassallo; j.vassallo@elsevier.com	**ISBN-13: 978-1-4160-5061-2**
	ISBN-10: 1-4160-5061-2

Dental Clinics of North America (ISSN 0011-8532) is published quarterly by Elsevier Inc., 360 Park Avenue South, New York, NY 10010-1710. Months of issue are January, April, July, and October. Business and Editorial Offices: 1600 John F. Kennedy Boulevard, Suite 1800, Philadelphia, PA 19103-2899. Customer Service Office: 6277 Sea Harbor Drive, Orlando, FL 32887-4800. Periodicals postage paid at New York, NY and additional mailing offices. Subscription prices are $171.00 per year (US individuals), $281.00 per year (US institutions), $83.00 per year (US students), $204.00 per year (Canadian individuals), $347.00 per year (Canadian institutions), $116.00 per year (Canadian students), $231.00 per year (international individuals), $347.00 per year (international institutions), and $116.00 per year (international students). International air speed delivery is included in all *Clinics* subscription prices. All prices are subject to change without notice. **POSTMASTER:** Send address changes to *Dental Clinics of North America*, Elsevier Periodicals Customer Service, 6277 Sea Harbor Drive, Orlando, FL 32887-4800. Customer Service: 1-800-654-2452 (US). From outside of the US, call 1-407-345-4000.

The Dental Clinics of North America is covered in *Index Medicus, Current Contents/Clinical Medicine, ISI/BIOMED* and *Clinahl*.

Printed in the United States of America.

GUEST EDITORS

LYLE D. ZARDIACKAS, PhD, FADM, Professor and Chair, Department of Biomedical Materials Science, University of Mississippi Medical Center School of Dentistry, Jackson, Mississippi

TRACY M. DELLINGER, DDS, MS, Associate Professor and Director, Advanced Education in General Dentistry Residency Program, Department of Advanced General Dentistry, University of Mississippi Medical Center School of Dentistry, Jackson, Mississippi

MARK LIVINGSTON, DDS, Associate Professor and Director, General Practice Residency Program, Department of Advanced General Dentistry, University of Mississippi Medical Center School of Dentistry, Jackson, Mississippi

CONTRIBUTORS

THOMAS H. ELLIS, PhD, Director of Research, Synchrotron Light Source, University of Saskatchewan, Saskatoon, Saskatchewan, Canada

JAMES G. FITCHIE, DMD, Professor, Care Planning and Restorative Sciences, University of Mississippi Medical Center School of Dentistry, Jackson, Mississippi

JEFFERSON GAMBLIN, BS, Fourth Year Dental Student, University of Mississippi Medical Center School of Dentistry, Jackson, Mississippi

R. SCOTT GATEWOOD, DMD, Associate Professor and Chair, Department of Endodontics, University of Mississippi School of Dentistry, Jackson, Mississippi

DANIEL A. GIVAN, DMD, PhD, Assistant Professor of Prosthodontics; and Assistant Director of Graduate Prosthodontics; and Director of Continuing Dental Education Graduate Prosthodontics, Department of Prosthodontics, University of Alabama at Birmingham School of Dentistry, Birmingham, Alabama

JASON A. GRIGGS, PhD, Associate Professor and Graduate Program Director, Department of Biomaterials Science, Baylor College of Dentistry, The Texas A&M University System Health Science Center, Dallas, Texas

EDWARD E. HILL, DDS, MS, Associate Professor, Department of Care Planning and Restorative Sciences, University of Mississippi Medical Center School of Dentistry, Jackson, Mississippi

PIA CHATERJEE KIRK, DDS, Assistant Professor, Care Planning and Restorative Sciences, University of Mississippi Medical Center School of Dentistry, Jackson, Mississippi

MARI KOIKE, DDS, PhD, Assistant Professor, Department of Biomaterials Science, Baylor College of Dentistry, The Texas A&M University System Health Science Center, Dallas, Texas

RICHARD J. MITCHELL, PhD, Associate Professor, Division of Restorative Dentistry, Department of Oral Health Practice, College of Dentistry, University of Kentucky, Lexington, Kentucky

TORU OKABE, PhD, Professor and Chair, Department of Biomaterials Science, Baylor College of Dentistry, The Texas A&M University System Health Science Center, Dallas, Texas

HARRY V. PRECHEUR, DMD, Associate Professor and Chair, Department of Oral and Maxillofacial Surgery and Pathology; and Associate Professor, Department of Surgery, Division of Plastic and Reconstructive Surgery, University of Mississippi Medical Center, Jackson, Mississippi

AARON D. PUCKETT, PhD, Professor, Care Planning and Restorative Sciences, University of Mississippi Medical Center School of Dentistry, Jackson, Mississippi

MICHAEL ROACH, MS, Instructor, Department of Biomedical Materials Research, University of Mississippi Medical Center School of Dentistry, Jackson, Mississippi

BARRY S. RUBEL, DMD, Associate Professor, Department of Care Planning and Restorative Sciences, University of Mississippi Medical Center School of Dentistry, Jackson, Mississippi

EDWARD SACHER, PhD, Department of Engineering Physics, École Polytechnique, Montréal, Québec, Canada

IVAN STANGEL, DMD, Scientific Director, BioMat Sciences, Bethesda, Maryland; Past Professor and Current Adjunct Professor, McGill University, Faculty of Dentistry, Montréal, Québec, Canada

KENNETH R. ST. JOHN, PhD, Associate Professor, Department of Biomedical Materials Science, University of Mississippi Medical Center School of Dentistry, Jackson, Mississippi

CONTENTS

The use of dental amalgam has declined, but in most of the world, amalgam is the most widely used and widely taught direct restorative material for load-bearing posterior restorations. There are few national regulations on the use of amalgam; however, there are several nations where few amalgam restorations are placed. Long-term studies have shown that under optimum conditions, posterior restorations of amalgam and resin composite last longer than reported previously and that amalgam restorations outlast composite restorations. In general practice settings, posterior amalgam and composite restorations both have lower longevities.

Precious alloys are an important material group in dentistry because of their ease of use, excellent compatibility, favorable mechanical and physical properties, and application in ceramometal bonding. Although new precious alloys have been introduced in the past decades, frequently because of economic pressure, gold-based alloys remain a popular choice. Researchers have suggested that alloys should be chosen based on an understanding of the alloy system, selection of proven alloys from quality manufacturers, and consideration of the requirements of a given clinical situation.

FORTHCOMING ISSUES

RECENT ISSUES

THE CLINICS ARE NOW AVAILABLE ONLINE!

Access your subscription at:
http://www.theclinics.com

THE DENTAL
CLINICS
OF NORTH AMERICA

Dent Clin N Am 51 (2007) xi–xii

Preface

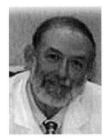
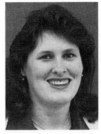
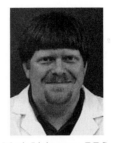

Lyle D. Zardiackas, PhD, FADM   Tracy M. Dellinger, DDS, MS   Mark Livingston, DDS
Guest Editors

The contents of the articles in this issue are meant to serve as a resource in the areas of dental materials applicable to dental practice with special emphasis on those areas that have seen major changes over the last two decades. The text is designed to give an overview of the science and state of the art areas presently used by dental students and practicing clinicians, rather than give a treatise on techniques or extensive discussion intended for the research scientist. Note the absence of information on biological materials with the exception of some used for bone grafting and other guided tissue materials. These biological systems are in their infancy of development and, in general, are not yet available for dental applications.

Basic information on specific materials is included in each article; however, the emphasis is, for the most part, focused on the clinical application, pitfalls, and failure of these materials to achieve their intended function. There are a number of excellent texts and research articles, many of which are cited in the article bibliographies. The reader who is interested in further study in any particular area is referred to the articles and books cited at the end of each article.

The hope is that this issue will not only serve as a reference for students, faculty, and practicing clinicians, but also that it will stimulate participation

doi:10.1016/j.cden.2007.05.001

in the research and development of superior materials. Clinical input is not only desirable; it is also necessary to optimize new product development.

Lyle D. Zardiackas, PhD, FADM
Professor and Chair
Department of Biomedical Materials Science, D528
University of Mississippi Medical Center School of Dentistry
2500 North State Street
Jackson, MS 39216, USA

E-mail address: lzardiackas@sod.umsmed.edu

Tracy M. Dellinger, DDS, MS
Associate Professor and Director
Advanced Education in General Dentistry Residency Program
Department of Advanced General Dentistry, D403-3
University of Mississippi Medical Center School of Dentistry
2500 North State Street
Jackson, MS 39216, USA

E-mail address: tdellinger@sod.umsmed.edu

Mark Livingston, DDS
Associate Professor and Director
General Practice Residency Program
Department of Advanced General Dentistry, D403-3
University of Mississippi Medical Center School of Dentistry
2500 North State Street
Jackson, MS 39216, USA

E-mail address: hlivingston@sod.umsmed.edu

ELSEVIER
SAUNDERS

THE DENTAL
CLINICS
OF NORTH AMERICA

Dent Clin N Am 51 (2007) 573–589

Posterior Amalgam Restorations—Usage, Regulation, and Longevity

Richard J. Mitchell, PhD[a],*, Mari Koike, DDS, PhD[b], Toru Okabe, PhD[b]

[a]*Division of Restorative Dentistry, Department of Oral Health Practice, College of Dentistry, University of Kentucky, D641 Medical Center, 800 Rose Street, Lexington, KY 40536-0297, USA*
[b]*Department of Biomaterials Science, Baylor College of Dentistry, The Texas A&M University System Health Science Center, 3302 Gaston Avenue, Dallas, TX 75246-2098, USA*

This article is a review of the literature on posterior amalgam restorations published during the period between 1996 and 2006. During this period, research interest on amalgam significantly declined. A Medline search of articles with "amalgam" in the title, "dental" anywhere, and the subject "dentistry" yielded 1054 citations (1.4% of all dental citations) between 1986 and 1995 but only 553 citations (0.81% of all dental citations) between 1996 and 2005. During the latter period, there were only two comprehensive reviews of the literature on dental amalgam, and both appeared early in the period [1,2]. Several articles referred to amalgam in the context of reviewing the advantages and disadvantages of alternative restorative materials, however [3–7].

Because there have been many recent reviews of amalgam biocompatibility [8–19] and the effects amalgam waste on the environment [20–22], this article focuses solely on amalgam restorations. Similarly, because recent reviews have focused on dental amalgam in primary teeth [23,24], the focus of this article is on amalgam in permanent teeth. Because of space limitations, an update on the metallurgical, physical, and mechanical properties of dental amalgam must await another venue.

The authors thank the National Institute of Dental Research of the US National Institutes of Health for more than two decades of support for the authors' research and that of other investigators who have greatly expanded our knowledge of this key dental material.

* Corresponding author.
E-mail address: rjm1@uky.edu (R.J. Mitchell).

Current usage

In 2004, Burke [25] reviewed trends in amalgam and composite usage around the world. The following discussion summarizes and updates Burke's excellent review.

North American dentists

Several reports suggested that the overall use of dental amalgam in the United States has declined significantly during the last decade [26–28]. In one state, the number of resin composite restorations exceeded the number of amalgam restorations in 1999 [27]. Amalgam continues to be the most widely used direct restorative material for posterior load-bearing restorations, however. In 1999, US dentists placed 71 million amalgam restorations compared with 46 million posterior resin composite restorations [28]. The number of posterior composites was up from 13 million in 1990; the number of amalgam restorations was down from 99 million placed in that year [28]. From 1990 to 1999, amalgam restorations declined from 88.4% to 60.6% of the sum of amalgam and posterior composite restorations.

North American dental schools

The best judgment of dental educators may be of interest. In a 1997 survey, 53 of 54 North American dental schools responding reported that they taught the use of resin composite to restore posterior teeth [29]. Thirty-seven percent of the schools devoted less than 5% of operative dentistry curriculum time to teaching class I and II composite restorations; 85% of the schools reported that they spent less than 20% of available curriculum time on these restorations. Only 30% of the surveyed schools taught three-surface class II posterior composites in molars. This study did not explicitly ask about the percentage of the operative curriculum devoted to teaching amalgam restoration. It is plausible that increased curriculum time for posterior composite restorations is an indicator of increased probability that composite will be selected over amalgam.

The trend was—and continues to be—toward greater emphasis on resin composite for posterior restorations. For example, in a 2005 survey, 68% of 47 US dental schools reported that they used resin composite for three-surface class II restorations [30]. This study also found that in 80% of US schools amalgam was taught first and that amalgam was used in 60% of the posterior restorations placed by students. A recent survey suggested that Canadian dental schools have a similar philosophy for direct posterior restorations [31]. Amalgam continues to be favored among Canadian educators: in all schools responding, amalgam and resin composite posterior restorations were taught, with either equal or greater emphasis being placed on amalgam [31].

European dentists

The use of amalgam in the United Kingdom is similar to that in the United States. In a 2001 survey of 654 British general dentists, 35% reported that they "sometimes" used resin composites in extensive load-bearing restorations in molar teeth [32]. Fifteen percent responded "often," and 1% responded "always" to this question. Presumably amalgam was used when resin composite was not. In a smaller survey, 30 UK dentists reported that 87% of class II and 67% of class I restorations were amalgam [33].

Amalgam is used less frequently in some Scandinavian countries. In 2002, Ylinen and Lofroth [34] reported that only 28% of Finnish dentists and 40% of Swedish dentists used amalgam. In the two other Scandinavian countries, however, amalgam was used by most dentists (88% of Danish dentists and 92% of Norwegian dentists). Use of amalgam is particularly low in Finland, where a 2000 survey returned by 548 dentists reported all the restorations they placed in a single working day. Amalgam accounted for only 8% of the class I restorations (resin composite: 80%) and 9% of the class II restorations (composite: 80%). When asked what material they would use to restore an occlusal lesion in the lower second molar in a 20-year-old patient, amalgam was the choice of 52.4% of 173 Danish dentists, 19.9% of 759 Norwegian dentists, and 2.9% of 923 Swedish dentists [35]. A 2005 report commissioned by the Swedish government found that amalgam fillings were no longer used in children and young people and that by weight amalgam made up only 6% of all Swedish fillings [36].

European dental schools

Responding to a 1997 survey, 100 of 104 (96%) European dental schools reported that they taught resin composites for class I restorations [37]. Seventy-nine percent of European schools taught three-surface class II posterior composites restorations; however, 56% of these schools devoted no more than 20% of the curriculum time for direct restorations to posterior composites. Only 38% of the surveyed schools taught three-surface class II posterior composites in molars. Overall, the European schools were similar to the North American schools in that amalgam was still taught for class I and II restorations, and at most schools, most of the curriculum time was spent on amalgam. A 2006 survey of dental schools in the United Kingdom suggested that the teaching of resin composite for posterior restoration continues to increase [38]. In this study, 9 of 15 schools (60%) reported that they taught three-surface class II resin composites.

The general trend is that amalgam continues to be taught in European dental schools. One dental school in the Netherlands has gradually reduced the amount of curriculum time devoted to dental amalgam as a restorative material [39]. In 2001, it stopped teaching amalgam altogether.

Dentists and dental schools in the rest of the world

Cross-sectional surveys of Australian dentists revealed that between 1984 and 1999, the use of amalgam gradually declined from 57.8% to 23.3% of all restorative services rendered [40]. In a 2002 survey of 560 randomly selected Australian dentists, 32% reported that they "sometimes" used resin composites in extensive load-bearing restorations in molar teeth [41]; 29% responded "often" and 12% responded "always" to this question. The former two categories revealed greater use of resin composite in Australia (41% "often" or "always") than in a similarly designed study conducted in the United Kingdom (16% "often" or "always") [32]. These data suggest a greater move away from amalgam in Australia than has been seen in Europe or the United States.

An even larger move away from amalgam has taken place in Japan. Unfortunately, there are only two reports of this in the English language literature, neither of which provides data [25,42]. Both articles report that amalgam is little used in general practice, which may be because of fear of mercury that gripped the Japanese public in the aftermath of the poisoning of inhabitants of Minamata and Niigata in the mid-1950s [42,43]. Victims had consumed methyl mercury–contaminated fish. Given the abandonment of amalgam, it is interesting that most Japanese dental schools do not view resin composite a suitable material in extensive class II restorations. In a 1997 survey, 25 of 27 Japanese dental schools taught resin composite for class I restorations, but less than 19% of the schools considered resin composite a suitable restorative material for three-surface class II restorations [44].

Data from the rest of the world are spotty. In some countries, dental amalgam may still be the major restorative material for load-bearing restorations. For example, a 1997 survey of 241 Jordanian dentists showed that dental amalgam was used for 88.8% of all class I and class II restorations [45,46]. In other countries, the trend is more like that seen in North American and Europe. For example, a 1999 survey revealed that 97% of 65 Brazilian schools surveyed considered resin composite suitable for class I restorations. Like faculty representing northern hemisphere dental schools, only 33% of Brazilian respondents considered resin composite suitable for three-surface class II restorations [47].

Regulation of amalgam use by governments

During the 1990s, anti-amalgam newsletters and Web sites reported that dental amalgam had been banned in Europe, especially in Germany and Sweden. Wahl [14] discussed and refuted these rumors. Similarly, after surveying regulatory agencies in ten countries, Burke [25] concluded that there "were few restrictions worldwide to the placement of dental amalgam." The tightest current restrictions seem to be in Denmark, where amalgam use is limited to molar teeth [25,48]. Sweden, Norway, Austria, and Germany recommend that amalgam restorations not be placed in pregnant women [25,48,49]. Germany also recommends that amalgam not be placed in patients with renal impairment [24]. Most of the other nations surveyed, including the United States, United Kingdom, Australia, Finland, and Ireland, have issued no recommendations for restrictions on amalgam use.

Although Sweden does not currently regulate amalgam, its national health system has not reimbursed dentists for amalgam restorations since 1999 [50]. This decision has greatly reduced use of amalgam. Sweden also has announced that its overall goal is to phase out use of mercury, including dental amalgam [46]. A 2004 report commissioned by the Swedish government confirmed this goal for mercury in general but recommended that dental amalgam be exempted from the general ban until December 31, 2008 [50]. A 2005 report commissioned by the Swedish government concluded that a phase out of dental amalgam restorations will not have a significant effect because amalgam is already used infrequently [36].

Longevity of amalgam restorations

When Mjor and colleagues [51] reviewed the longevity of posterior restorations in 1990, it was evident that median survival times of amalgam restorations in posterior teeth varied greatly among studies. Sixteen years later, restoration longevity data can appear just as chaotic. For example, in 2004, Manhard and colleagues [52] reviewed clinical studies of various restorative materials placed in posterior teeth, including 41 studies of amalgams and 50 studies of resin composites (see also their earlier reviews [53,54]). They found that the ranges of annual failure rates were wide: 0 to 7.4% for amalgams and 0 to 9.0% for composite. From these studies they calculated mean failure annual rates of 3% (standard deviation, 1.9%) for amalgams and 2.2% (standard deviation, 2%) for posterior composites [52]. This does not mean that composites fared better than amalgams; the two failure rates are not statistically different. One might erroneously conclude, however, that posterior composite restorations would be at least as successful in posterior restorations as amalgam.

Manhard and colleagues concede that it is "problematic to directly compare different studies from different authors," but they are not explicit about some of the pitfalls of combining data from different studies [52]. For example, as Mackert and Wahl [5] noted, many of the cited studies are relatively short-term (≤5 years). Such studies are biased because they exclude failure modes that occur more frequently later in a restoration's life (marginal degradation, secondary caries, bulk fracture, and tooth fracture) [51]. Manhard and Hickel's mean annual failure rates combine data from two different types of studies: (1) controlled longitudinal clinical trials, in which restorations are placed and maintained under conditions that are favorable to longevity and (2) uncontrolled studies in general practice, in which restorations have been placed and maintained under conditions less favorable to longevity. The former shows whether a restorative material has the potential to be used successfully and the latter shows whether that potential is actually being achieved [51,55,56]. To meaningfully compare the longevity of posterior amalgam and composite restorations, one must be sure that the restorations to be compared have been studied under similar conditions.

Longitudinal studies

The best way to estimate the longevity of restorations is to conduct longitudinal trials [57]. Unfortunately, longitudinal studies are expensive, require long-term commitment of personnel and other resources, and may be plagued by loss of patients [51,58]. As a result, few studies of dental restorative materials have continued long enough to obtain long-term data. Short-term studies may underreport types of failure (eg, secondary caries and fatigue fracture) that are likely to become more important after many years in vivo. When new failure mechanisms become operative late in a restoration's life, short-term studies overestimate restoration longevity [59].

In the following sections and in the accompanying tables, longitudinal studies in which restorations have been followed for at least 8 years are emphasized. To help the reader compare results, failure rates have been extrapolated to median survival times. When median survival times have been determined from life tables, it is noted in the tables. It should be cautioned, however, that extrapolated data, even from long-term studies, assume that past performance will predict future behavior. The future is not certain: the failure rate may speed up as new failure mechanisms become operative as time progresses, or conversely, the failure rate may slow as early failures eliminate the restorations most at risk of failure from the study population.

Longitudinal studies in optimum setting

Studies conducted in these settings, typically dental schools, tend to show a material's durability under optimum conditions [57,60]. Patients are often dentally aware. They are often dental students, dental school staff, or conscientious patients who are judged especially likely to return for recall appointments. Typically, operator variability is reduced by using only a few (usually less than six) dentists. These dentists are often teaching staff who are well calibrated and likely to adhere closely to study protocols. Importantly, these dentists seldom function under tight time constraints like those in private practice.

Several 5- to 8-year longitudinal studies of posterior amalgam restorations appeared during the 1980s. The results of these studies suggested that in optimum settings dental amalgam restorations might last much longer than previously thought. For example, amalgam restorations in a set of studies reviewed by Letzel and colleagues [61] had median survival times of

11.4 to 87.5 years for low-copper amalgams and between 19.2 and more than 150 years for high-copper amalgam restorations (Table 1) [62–66]. During the last 15 years, longitudinal studies of even longer duration have appeared. In longitudinal prospective trials, class I and II amalgam restorations were found to have median survival times of 57.5 years [67], 65.8 years [61], and 69 years [68].

Table 1
Longitudinal studies of amalgam restorations in posterior teeth of at least 8 years' duration (1990–2006)

Authors	Year	Study type[a]	Study setting[b]	Study duration (y)	No. of dentists	No. of restorations	Median survival time (y)	Survival estimate method[c]
Studies of class I and II amalgam restorations								
Osborne & Norman [67]	1990	P	+	13	1	181	57.5	A
Letzel et al [61]	1997	P	+	5–15	7	3244	65.8	E
Collins et al [68]	1998	P	++	8	1	53	69.0	A
Dawson & Smales [69][d]	1992	R	++++	0–17	many	1345	14.4	B
Lucarotti et al [70][d]	2005	R	++++	0–12	many	76,418	11.9	E
Bjertness & Sonyu [71][d]	1990	R	++	0–17	4	782	44.7	F
Hawthorne & Smales [72][d]	1997	R	+++	mean 25	20	1728	22.5	B
Smales [73][d]	1991	P	++	8–10	many	1476	62.5	F
Class II restorations only								
Gruythuysen et al [74]	1996	P	+	15	3	1213	44.1	A
Jokstad & Mjor [75]	1991	P	++	9.5	7	469	25.0	E
Smales [76]	1991	P	++	15	many	664	27.2	F
Lucarotti et al [70]—distal-occlusal & mesial-occlusal restorations	2005	R	++++	0–12	many	16,680	9.8	E
Lucarotti et al [70]—mesial-occlusal-distal restorations	2005	R	++++	0–12	many	147,087	8.8	E

[a] P, prospective; R, retrospective.

[b] +, controlled; ++, closer to controlled; +++, closer to general practice; ++++, general practice.

[c] A, Survival time extrapolated from percentage of restorations surviving at end of study. B, Survival time is taken directly from a life table. C, Survival time is extrapolated from a life table. D, Survival time is taken directly from survival plots calculated by the Kaplan-Meier method. E, Survival time is extrapolated from survival plots calculated by the Kaplan-Meier method. F, Survival time is extrapolated from actuarial life tables.

[d] Some classes III and V but predominantly classes I and II.

Longitudinal studies in general practice settings

Two relatively recent longitudinal studies have shown that amalgam restorations do not survive as long in general practice settings as in clinical trials. The first study was a retrospective longitudinal analysis of all types of amalgam restorations placed in Australian Air Force clinic patients between 1972 and 1988 [69]. They found a median survival time of just 14.4 years. The sites in which the restorations were placed were not reported. It is presumed that most of the restorations were class I or II. Class III and V restorations included in this study would most likely have increased survival time.

The second report of the survival of amalgam restorations placed in general practices appeared recently. In a retrospective longitudinal study, Lucarotti and colleagues [70] used insurance payment records to follow a large number of restorations placed by the General Dental Service of the United Kingdom between 1990 and 2001. The median survival time of single surface amalgam restorations (presumably mostly class I restorations) was 11.9 years.

Longer survival times are sometimes reported for studies conducted in what seems to be general practice populations. When case selection is scrutinized, however, one concludes that the data are not typical of general practices. For example, Bjertness and Sonju [71] conducted a retrospective longitudinal study of records from the general practices of six Norwegian dentists. This 17-year study yielded a 44.7-year median survival time for amalgams of unknown composition. The survival time may have been increased by the use of a study population that was limited to patients who returned annually for examination. Such conscientiousness suggests that the selected patients have a high dental awareness. Patient oral hygiene may have been better than is typical in general practice populations. That four of the dentists worked part time at a dental school also may have increased the durability.

As was the case in Bjertness and Sonju's [71] study, in their retrospective study of restoration longevity in three Australian practices, Hawthorne and Smales [72] selected patients who had "a continuous attendance history." They found a median survival time of 22.5 years. The selection of highly conscientious patients may have increased survival time. On the other hand, more than 64% of the restorations were class II amalgams. The predominance of class II amalgam in the sample may explain why the median survival time was less than that found by Bjertness and Sonju. Note, however, that Bjertness and Sonju did not report the distribution of restorations by class, so one does not know for sure that one study is more class II–rich than the other.

Smales [73] reported on the 10-year durability of a set of amalgam restorations placed in an Australian dental school clinic by dental students and staff. The study setting was neither a general practice nor a well-controlled clinical trial. The median survival time of the amalgams restorations in this setting was 62.5 years. This long durability suggests that the dental school setting may be closer to the optimum setting of a controlled clinical trial than it is to a general practice setting.

Longitudinal studies of class II restorations

Under optimum conditions, class I and II amalgam restorations are found to have median survival times between 57 and 70 years. As might be expected, similar trials of just class II restorations yield shorter survival times. In one such study, the median survival time was 44.1 years (Table 1) [74]. In another study, median survival time was 25 years [75]. The survival time of the latter may have been reduced by two of the six operators who placed their restorations in general practice settings. A study under slightly less than optimum conditions gave similar results. In a study conducted in an Australian dental hospital, where restorations were placed by a large number of student and staff dentists, Smales [76] found a medium survival time of 27.6 years. These survival times are longer than found general practice settings, however. In a large retrospective longitudinal study by Lucarotti and colleagues [70], class II amalgams placed in general practices in the United Kingdom were found to have median survival times of 9.8 years for distal-occlusal and mesial-occlusal restorations and 8.8 years for mesial-distal-occlusal restorations.

Longitudinal studies of extensive posterior restorations

Restorations in which one or more cusp has been restored with amalgam exhibit even shorter survival times. Table 2 provides some details of longitudinal studies of such restorations. Three prospective longitudinal studies were conducted in optimum settings; two are in good agreement. In one study, the median survival time was found to be 14.9 years [77]. In a second study, the median survival time was found to be 12.5 years for molars with all cusps covered and 14.5 years for molars with only partial cusp coverage [78]. In a third study, however, a longer median survival time was found: 27.4 years for amalgams with a least one cusp covered with amalgam [76]. In this last study, the investigator also reported that the survival time for complex amalgams was not significantly different than class II amalgam restorations in the same patient pool [76]. This observation suggested that the extensive amalgams may have included fewer cusps than other studies.

Three retrospective longitudinal studies of extensive amalgam in general practice settings also have been conducted. In one study, investigators sampled records from US Air Force dental clinics and found a median survival time of 11.5 years [79]. In a second study, investigators examined records of an HMO based in Oregon [80]. They found a median survival time of 8.9 years for four-surface amalgam restorations and a median time of 7.1 years for five-surface amalgam restorations. Investigators in a third study found a longer median survival time of 14.4 years [81]. These restorations were

Table 2

Longitudinal studies of extensive amalgam restorations in posterior teeth of at least 5 years' duration (1988–2006)

Authors	Year	Study type[a]	Study setting[b]	Study duration (y)	No. of dentists	No. of restorations	Median survival time (y)	Survival estimate method[c]
Plasmans et al [77]	1998	P	+	8.3	3	300	14.9	C
Van Nieuwenhuysen et al [78] molars; complete coverage	2003	P	+	1–17	1	226	12.5	D
Van Nieuwenhuysen et al [78] molars; partial coverage	2003	P	+	1–17	1	434	14.5	D
Smales [76] with cusp coverage	1991	P	++	15	many	124	27.4	F
Smales [76] without cusp coverage	1991	P	++	15	many	664	27.2	F
Robbins & Summitt [79]	1988	R	++++	1–20	many	171	11.5	B
Martin & Bader [80] 4-surface amalgam	1997	R	++++	5	74	2038	8.9	A
Martin & Bader [80] 5-surface amalgam	1997	R	++++	5	74	1626	7.1	A
Smales & Hawthorne [81]	1997	R	++	mean 25	20	160	14.4	C

[a] P, prospective; R, retrospective.

[b] +, controlled; ++, closer to controlled; +++, closer to general practice ++++, general practice.

[c] A, Survival time extrapolated from percentage of restoration surviving at end of study. B, Survival time is taken directly from a life table. C, Survival time is extrapolated from a life table. D, Survival time is taken directly from survival plots calculated by the Kaplan-Meier method. E, Survival time is extrapolated from survival plots calculated by the Kaplan-Meier method. F, Survival time is extrapolated from actuarial life tables.

from three Australian general practices. One hundred patients who had been in continuous attendance for at least 12 years were selected. The selection of highly motivated patients and the use of a small number of dentists may have combined to produce a longer survival time than is typical in general practice.

For comparison: longitudinal studies of resin composite restoration in posterior teeth

How does the longevity of posterior composite compare with that of amalgam restorations? Table 3 summarizes details of several long-term longitudinal studies of posterior resin composite restorations that have been reported during the last 15 years. In studies conducted under "optimum" conditions, median survival times for posterior composite restorations made with particular brands of composite were 44.3 [82], 24.4 [68], 26 [68], 43 [68], 19.4 [83], and 20.2 [84] years. The combined median survival

Table 3
Longitudinal studies of resin composite restorations in posterior teeth of at least 5 years' duration (1998–2006)

Authors	Year	Study type[a]	Study setting[b]	Study duration (y)	No. of dentists	No. of restorations	Median survival time (y)	Survival estimate method[c]
Lundin & Koch [82], RC1[d]	1999	P	+	10	2	65	15.3	A
Lundin & Koch [82], RC2	1999	P	+	10	2	72	32.7	A
Collins et al [68], RC3	1998	P	+	8	1	55	24.4	A
Collins et al [68], RC4	1998	P	+	8	1	52	26.0	A
Collins et al [68], RC5	1998	P	+	8	1	54	43.0	A
Gaengler et al [83], RC6	2001	P	+	10	4	194	19.4	A
van Dijken [84], RC7	2000	P	+	11	1	34	20.2	A
Raskin et al [87], RC1	1999	P	+	10	1	100	8.0	A
Wilder et al [85], 4 RCs	1999	P	+	17	2	100	35.4	A
Pallesen & Qvist [86], 2RCs	2003	P	+	11	1	56	34.4	A
da Rosa Rodolpho et al [88]	2006	P	+++	17	1	282	approximately 16	D
Kohler et al [90], RC8 & RC9	2000	P	++++	5	many	63	9.1	A
Opdam et al [89], RC8	2004	R	+++	5	many	609	19.2	A

[a] P, prospective; R, retrospective.

[b] +, controlled; ++, closer to controlled; +++, closer to general practice ++++, general practice.

[c] A, Survival time extrapolated from percentage of restoration surviving at end of study. B, Survival time is taken directly from a life table. C, Survival time is extrapolated from a life table. D, Survival time is taken directly from survival plots calculated by the Kaplan-Meier method. E, Survival time is extrapolated from survival plots calculated by the Kaplan-Meier method. F, Survival time is extrapolated from actuarial life tables.

[d] RC, resin composite. (See articles for brand names and manufacturers.)

time of restorations made from four brands of ultraviolet-cured resin composites was 35.4 years [85]. The combined median survival time of posterior restorations made from two other brands of resin composite was 44.4 years [86]. These values suggested that posterior resin composite restorations can potentially be durable. These survival times fall considerably short of the 57- to 90-year range of median survival times found for posterior amalgam restorations under similar "optimum" conditions.

Note that one brand of resin composite studied under optimum conditions exhibited considerably shorter median survival times (15.3 [82] and 8.0 [87] years) than the other composites. This material seems to be of lower quality than other resin composites currently on the market. In studies in which more than one brand of resin composite was evaluated, survival time often varied significantly by brand [68,82].

One of the studies included in Table 3, that of Collins and colleagues [68], followed posterior restorations made with three brands of resin composites and one brand of amalgam. The median survival time for the amalgam restorations was 69 years—1.6 times that of the best of the resin composite restorations in the same study. The amalgam restorations survived approximately 2.6 times as long as restorations made with the other two brands of resin composite.

One would like to be able to compare the longevity of posterior amalgam and composite restorations in general practice settings. Recall that in general practice, posterior amalgam restorations are found to have median survival times of 8 to 15 years. Unfortunately, there has been only one report of a long-term general practice–based longitudinal study of posterior composite restorations. This study, which followed restorations placed in a Brazilian general practice for 17 years, was recently reported by da Rosa Rodolpho and colleagues [88]. They found that the median survival time for posterior composite restorations was approximately 16 years. Based on this result, one is tempted to conclude that the performance of posterior composite restorations is better than that of amalgam restorations in general practice settings. Note, however, that the survival time may have been improved by using a single motivated clinician, a practice that emphasized oral hygiene, and the selection of highly motivated patients who returned annually for appointments.

Because of the dearth of long-term general practice–based longitudinal data on posterior composite restorations, one is forced to consider results from briefer studies. Two such studies are included in Table 3. Opdam and colleagues [89] followed class I and II resin composites that were placed by supervised student dentists in a Dutch dental school. They found a median survival time of 19.2 years. This last result may have been positively biased by a strictly supervised, unhurried dental school setting. The other study was conducted under conditions that were closer to general practice settings. Kohler and colleagues [90] followed class II resin composites that were placed by a large number of loosely calibrated dentists in three Swedish public health clinics. After 5 years, they found a median survival time of 9.1 years.

Relatively brief studies, such as those discussed previously, fail to detect accelerated failures rates caused by failure mechanisms that become important after years in the mouth. It is interesting to note that in the 17-year general practice study of da Rosa Rodolpho and colleagues [88], two brands of resin composite exhibit a relatively low failure rate (5%) at 10 years but that after 10 years, the failure rate increases rapidly: 14% at 12 years, 40% at 15 years, and 72% at 17 years. Based on a 5% failure rate at 10 years, the restorations in the study by da Rosa Rudolpho and colleagues would have had an extrapolated median survival time of 100 years. It is likely that many of the studies of posterior restorations, both amalgam and composite, in which the median survival time exceeds the study duration significantly overestimate survival time.

Summary

The percentage of posterior teeth that are restored with resin composite continues to grow. In most of the world, however, dental amalgam remains the most widely used material for load-bearing restorations in posterior teeth. In the United States, amalgam is used for approximately 60% of all direct posterior restorations. Dental schools throughout the world continue to teach amalgam as the material of choice for large and complex posterior restorations. To date, no nation has outlawed the use of amalgam. Several nations have cautioned dentists against placing amalgam restorations in pregnant women, and Denmark limits amalgam to molar teeth. Few amalgam restorations are placed in Japan, Finland, and Sweden, however. As part of its plan to ban all mercury-containing products, Sweden is scheduled to ban dental amalgam by the end of 2008. Posterior amalgam restorations are more widely used and taught in the United States, Canada, and the United Kingdom than in Europe, Scandinavia, and Australia.

Long-term data from longitudinal studies that have become available over the last 10 years have made possible a reassessment of the durability of amalgam restorations in posterior teeth. The longevity of amalgam restorations depends on the setting in which they are placed. Studies conducted in general practices produced median survival times for posterior amalgam restorations of 7 to 15 years. Survival times for larger, more complex restorations fall within the lower end of this range. Studies conducted in "optimum settings" (typically in dental schools, in which a limited number of calibrated dentists working under few time constraints place restorations in motivated patients) revealed median survival times of 55 to 70 years. Comparable studies of posterior resin composites placed in optimum settings revealed median survival times of 20 to 45 years. Studies in optimum settings suggest that the potential survival time of amalgam and resin composite in posterior teeth is longer than had been thought and that under these conditions, amalgam outlasts composite. Unfortunately, no long-term studies of posterior resin composites have been conducted in general practice settings. Relatively short-term studies suggest that the median survival time of posterior resin composite studies may be less than 10 years. Long-term studies of resin composite restorations placed in general practice settings are badly needed.

References

[1] Berry TG, Summitt JB, Chung AK, et al. Amalgam at the new millennium. J Am Dent Assoc 1998;129(11):1547–56.
[2] Dunne SM, Gainsford ID, Wilson NH. Current materials and techniques for direct restorations in posterior teeth. Part 1: silver amalgam. Int Dent J 1997;47(3):123–36.
[3] Baghdadi ZD. Preservation-based approaches to restore posterior teeth with amalgam, resin or a combination of materials. Am J Dent 2002;15(1):54–65.
[4] Eley BM. The future of dental amalgam: a review of the literature. Part 7: possible alternative materials to amalgam for the restoration of posterior teeth. Br Dent J 1997;183(1):11–4.
[5] Mackert JR Jr, Wahl MJ. Are there acceptable alternatives to amalgam? J Calif Dent Assoc 2004;32(7):601–10.
[6] Roulet JF. Benefits and disadvantages of tooth-coloured alternatives to amalgam. J Dent 1997;25(6):459–73.
[7] Lutz F, Krejci I. Resin composites in the post-amalgam age. Compend Contin Educ Dent 1999;20(12):1138–44, 1146, 1148.
[8] Eley BM. The future of dental amalgam: a review of the literature. Part 2: mercury exposure in dental practice. Br Dent J 1997;182(8):293–7.
[9] Eley BM. The future of dental amalgam: a review of the literature. Part 1: dental amalgam structure and corrosion. Br Dent J 1997;182(7):247–9.
[10] Eley BM. The future of dental amalgam: a review of the literature. Part 3: mercury exposure from amalgam restorations in dental patients. Br Dent J 1997;182(9):333–8.
[11] Eley BM. The future of dental amalgam: a review of the literature. Part 4: mercury exposure hazards and risk assessment. Br Dent J 1997;182(10):373–81.
[12] Eley BM. The future of dental amalgam: a review of the literature. Part 5: mercury in the urine, blood and body organs from amalgam fillings. Br Dent J 1997;182(11):413–7.
[13] Eley BM. The future of dental amalgam: a review of the literature. Part 6: possible harmful effects of mercury from dental amalgam. Br Dent J 1997;182(12):455–9.
[14] Wahl MJ. Amalgam: resurrection and redemption. Part 1: the clinical and legal mythology of anti-amalgam. Quintessence Int 2001;32(7):525–35.
[15] Wahl MJ. Amalgam: resurrection and redemption. Part 2: the medical mythology of anti-amalgam. Quintessence Int 2001;32(9):696–710.
[16] Yip HK, Li DK, Yau DC. Dental amalgam and human health. Int Dent J 2003;53(6):464–8.
[17] Mutter J, Naumann J, Sadaghiani C, et al. Amalgam studies: disregarding basic principles of mercury toxicity. Int J Hyg Environ Health 2004;207(4):391–7.
[18] Brownawell AM, Berent S, Brent RL, et al. The potential adverse health effects of dental amalgam. Toxicol Rev 2005;24(1):1–10.
[19] Mitchell RJ, Osborne PB, Haubenreich JE. Dental amalgam restorations: daily mercury dose and biocompatibility. J Long Term Eff Med Implants 2005;15(6):709–21.
[20] Kao RT, Dault S, Pichay T. Understanding the mercury reduction issue: the impact of mercury on the environment and human health. J Calif Dent Assoc 2004;32(7):574–9.
[21] Horsted Bindslev P. Amalgam toxicity: environmental and occupational hazards. J Dent 2004;32(5):359–65.
[22] Johnson WJ, Pichay TJ. Dentistry, amalgam, and pollution prevention. J Calif Dent Assoc 2001;29(7):509–17.
[23] Osborne JW, Summitt JB, Roberts HW. The use of dental amalgam in pediatric dentistry: review of the literature. Pediatr Dent 2002;24(5):439–47.
[24] Fuks AB. The use of amalgam in pediatric dentistry. Pediatr Dent 2002;24(5):448–55.
[25] Burke FJ. Amalgam to tooth-coloured materials: implications for clinical practice and dental education. Governmental restrictions and amalgam-usage survey results. J Dent 2004;32(5):343–50.
[26] del Aguila MA, Anderson M, Porterfield D, et al. Patterns of oral care in a Washington state dental service population. J Am Dent Assoc 2002;133(3):343–51.

[27] Bogacki RE, Hunt RJ, del Aguila M, et al. Survival analysis of posterior restorations using an insurance claims database. Oper Dent 2002;27(5):488–92.

[28] Berthold M. Restoratives trend data shows shift in use of materials. ADA News 2002;33 1, 10, 11.

[29] Mjor IA, Wilson NH. Teaching class I and class II direct composite restorations: results of a survey of dental schools. J Am Dent Assoc 1998;129(10):1415–21.

[30] Lynch CD, McConnell RJ, Wilson NH. Teaching the placement of posterior resin-based composite restorations in U.S. dental schools. J Am Dent Assoc 2006;137(5):619–25.

[31] McComb D. Class I and class II silver amalgam and resin composite posterior restorations: teaching approaches in Canadian faculties of dentistry. J Can Dent Assoc 2005;71(6):405–6.

[32] Burke FJ, McHugh S, Hall AC, et al. Amalgam and composite use in UK general dental practice in 2001. Br Dent J 2003;194(11):613–8.

[33] Burke FJ, Wilson NH, Cheung SW, et al. Influence of patient factors on age of restorations at failure and reasons for their placement and replacement. J Dent 2001;29(5):317–24.

[34] Ylinen K, Lofroth G. Nordic dentists' knowledge and attitudes on dental amalgam from health and environmental perspectives. Acta Odontol Scand 2002;60(5):315–20.

[35] Espelid I, Tveit AB, Mejare I, et al. Restorative treatment decisions on occlusal caries in Scandinavia. Acta Odontol Scand 2001;59(1):21–7.

[36] Swedish National Chemical Inspectorate: Mercury-free dental fillings: phase-out of amalgam in Sweden. KEMI Report Nr 9/05. Sundbyberg, Sweden: Swedish National Chemical Inspectorate; 2005. p. 1–14.

[37] Wilson NH, Mjor IA. The teaching of class I and class II direct composite restorations in European dental schools. J Dent 2000;28(1):15–21.

[38] Lynch CD, McConnell RJ, Wilson NH. Teaching of posterior composite resin restorations in undergraduate dental schools in Ireland and the United Kingdom. Eur J Dent Educ 2006; 10(1):38–43.

[39] Roeters FJ, Opdam NJ, Loomans BA. The amalgam-free dental school. J Dent 2004;32(5): 371–7.

[40] Brennan DS, Spencer AJ. Restorative service trends in private general practice in Australia: 1983–1999. J Dent 2003;31(2):143–51.

[41] Burke FJ, McHugh S, Randall RC, et al. Direct restorative materials use in Australia in 2002. Aust Dent J 2004;49(4):185–91.

[42] Qualtrough AJ, Piddock V. Dental education in Japan. Br Dent J 1993;174(3):111–2.

[43] Harada M. Minamata disease: methylmercury poisoning in Japan caused by environmental pollution. Crit Rev Toxicol 1995;25(1):1–24.

[44] Fukushima M, Iwaku M, Setcos JC, et al. Teaching of posterior composite restorations in Japanese dental schools. Int Dent J 2000;50(6):407–11.

[45] AlNegrish AR. Composite resin restorations: a cross-sectional survey of placement and replacement in Jordan. Int Dent J 2002;52(6):461–8.

[46] AlNegrish AR. Reasons for placement and replacement of amalgam restorations in Jordan. Int Dent J 2001;51(2):109–15.

[47] Gordan VV, Mjor IA, Veiga Filho LC, et al. Teaching of posterior resin-based composite restorations in Brazilian dental schools. Quintessence Int 2000;31(10):735–40.

[48] UNEP Chemicals. Global mercury assessment. Geneva, Switzerland: United Nations Environment Programme; 2002. p. 266.

[49] Working Group on Dental Amalgam. Dental amalgam and alternative restorative materials. US Department of Health and Human Services, Public Health Service; 1997. Available at: http://www.health.gov/environment/amalgam2/National.html. Accessed May 17, 2007.

[50] Swedish National Chemical Inspectorate. Mercury: investigation of a general ban. KEMI Report No 4/04. Sundyberg, Sweden: Swedish National Chemical Inspectorate; 2004. p. 31–43.

[51] Mjor IA, Jokstad A, Qvist V. Longevity of posterior restorations. Int Dent J 1990;40(1): 11–7.

[52] Manhart J, Chen H, Hamm G, et al. Buonocore Memorial Lecture: review of the clinical survival of direct and indirect restorations in posterior teeth of the permanent dentition. Oper Dent 2004;29(5):481–508.

[53] Hickel R, Manhart J, Garcia Godoy F. Clinical results and new developments of direct posterior restorations. Am J Dent 2000;13(Spec No):41d–54d.

[54] Hickel R, Manhart J. Longevity of restorations in posterior teeth and reasons for failure. J Adhes Dent 2001;3(1):45–64.

[55] Burke FJ. Evaluating restorative materials and procedures in dental practice. Adv Dent Res 2005;18(3):46–9.

[56] Mjor IA. The basis for everyday real-life operative dentistry. Oper Dent 2001;26(5): 521–4.

[57] Wilson NH. The evaluation of materials: relationships between laboratory investigations and clinical studies. Oper Dent 1990;15(4):149–55.

[58] Hondrum SO. The longevity of resin-based composite restorations in posterior teeth. Gen Dent 2000;48(4):398–404.

[59] Davies JA. Dental restoration longevity: a critique of the life table method of analysis. Community Dent Oral Epidemiol 1987;15(4):202–4.

[60] Wilson NH, Mjor IA. Practice-based research: importance, challenges and prospects. A personal view. Prim Dent Care 1997;4(1):5–6.

[61] Letzel H, van't Hof MA, Marshall GW, et al. The influence of the amalgam alloy on the survival of amalgam restorations: a secondary analysis of multiple controlled clinical trials. J Dent Res 1997;76(11):1787–98.

[62] Osborne JW, Binon PP, Gale EN. Dental amalgam: clinical behavior up to eight years. Oper Dent 1980;5(1):24–8.

[63] Doglia R, Herr P, Holz J, et al. Clinical evaluation of four amalgam alloys: a five-year report. J Prosthet Dent 1986;56(4):406–15.

[64] van Dijken JW. A six year follow-up of three dental alloy restorations with different copper contents. Swed Dent J 1991;15(6):259–64.

[65] Letzel H. Survival rates and reasons for failure of posterior composite restorations in multicentre clinical trial. J Dent 1989;17(Suppl 1):S10–7 [discussion: S26–18].

[66] Letzel H, van't Hof MA, Vrijhoef MM, et al. A controlled clinical study of amalgam restorations: survival, failures, and causes of failure. Dent Mater 1989;5(2):115–21.

[67] Osborne JW, Norman RD. 13-year clinical assessment of 10 amalgam alloys. Dent Mater 1990;6(3):189–94.

[68] Collins CJ, Bryant RW, Hodge KL. A clinical evaluation of posterior composite resin restorations: 8-year findings. J Dent 1998;26(4):311–7.

[69] Dawson AS, Smales RJ. Restoration longevity in an Australian defence force population. Aust Dent J 1992;37(3):196–200.

[70] Lucarotti PS, Holder RL, Burke FJ. Outcome of direct restorations placed within the general dental services in England and Wales (Part 1): variation by type of restoration and re-intervention. J Dent 2005;33(10):805–15.

[71] Bjertness E, Sonju T. Survival analysis of amalgam restorations in long-term recall patients. Acta Odontol Scand 1990;48(2):93–7.

[72] Hawthorne WS, Smales RJ. Factors influencing long-term restoration survival in three private dental practices in Adelaide. Aust Dent J 1997;42(1):59–63.

[73] Smales RJ. Longevity of low- and high-copper amalgams analyzed by preparation class, tooth site, patient age, and operator. Oper Dent 1991;16(5):162–8.

[74] Gruythuysen RJ, Kreulen CM, Tobi H, et al. 15-year evaluation of class II amalgam restorations. Community Dent Oral Epidemiol 1996;24(3):207–10.

[75] Jokstad A, Mjor IA. Analyses of long-term clinical behavior of class-II amalgam restorations. Acta Odontol Scand 1991;49(1):47–63.

[76] Smales RJ. Longevity of cusp-covered amalgams: survivals after 15 years. Oper Dent 1991; 16(1):17–20.

[77] Plasmans PJ, Creugers NH, Mulder J. Long-term survival of extensive amalgam restorations. J Dent Res 1998;77(3):453–60.

[78] Van Nieuwenhuysen JP, D'Hoore W, Carvalho J, et al. Long-term evaluation of extensive restorations in permanent teeth. J Dent 2003;31(6):395–405.

[79] Robbins JW, Summitt JB. Longevity of complex amalgam restorations. Oper Dent 1988; 13(2):54–7.

[80] Martin JA, Bader JD. Five-year treatment outcomes for teeth with large amalgams and crowns. Oper Dent 1997;22(2):72–8.

[81] Smales RJ, Hawthorne WS. Long-term survival of extensive amalgams and posterior crowns. J Dent 1997;25(3–4):225–7.

[82] Lundin SA, Koch G. Class I and II posterior composite resin restorations after 5 and 10 years. Swed Dent J 1999;23(5–6):165–71.

[83] Gaengler P, Hoyer I, Montag R. Clinical evaluation of posterior composite restorations: the 10-year report. J Adhes Dent 2001;3(2):185–94.

[84] van Dijken JW. Direct resin composite inlays/onlays: an 11 year follow-up. J Dent 2000; 28(5):299–306.

[85] Wilder AD Jr, May KN Jr, Bayne SC, et al. Seventeen-year clinical study of ultraviolet-cured posterior composite class I and II restorations. J Esthet Dent 1999;11(3):135–42.

[86] Pallesen U, Qvist V. Composite resin fillings and inlays: an 11-year evaluation. Clin Oral Investig 2003;7(2):71–9.

[87] Raskin A, Michotte Theall B, Vreven J, et al. Clinical evaluation of a posterior composite 10-year report. J Dent 1999;27(1):13–9.

[88] da Rosa Rodolpho PA, Cenci MS, Donassollo TA, et al. A clinical evaluation of posterior composite restorations: 17-year findings. J Dent 2006;34(7):427–35.

[89] Opdam NJ, Loomans BA, Roeters FJ, et al. Five-year clinical performance of posterior resin composite restorations placed by dental students. J Dent 2004;32(5):379–83.

[90] Kohler B, Rasmusson CG, Odman P. A five-year clinical evaluation of class II composite resin restorations. J Dent 2000;28(2):111–6.

Precious Metals in Dentistry

Daniel A. Givan, DMD, PhD

*Department of Prosthodontics, University of Alabama at Birmingham School of Dentistry,
1530 3rd Avenue South, Birmingham, AL 35294-0007, USA*

Metals may be classified in two basic groups: ferrous and nonferrous. Ferrous metals contain iron and include metals such as steel. Nonferrous metals refer to noble metals, base metals, and light metals. Noble metals include gold and the platinum group, which contains platinum, palladium, ruthenium, rhodium, iridium, and osmium. They are characterized by good chemical stability to oxidation and resistance to corrosion and tarnish. Noble metals are often referred to as precious metals because of their relative high cost. Although silver is also considered to be a precious metal, poor resistance to corrosion and tarnish preclude it from being noble. Light metals, such as titanium, are characterized by their low density, whereas base metals include nickel, cobalt, and other heavy metals.

Most metals used in dentistry are in the form of alloys, or mixtures of one or more metal. Alloys are advantageous compared with pure metals in physical and mechanical properties because of engineering the optimum influence from each constituent. For example, pure gold is ductile, malleable, and soft, which is not desirable for prosthetic applications such as crowns. Introduction of additional metals into the gold increases the usefulness by altering the properties of the alloy through creation of solid solutions, precipitates, and multiple phases or by controlling grain size [1]. The addition of only 10% copper to gold results in a fourfold increase in tensile strength and similar increase in hardness [2]. The amount of gold in an alloy may be expressed by the number of carats or fineness of gold (Table 1). Pure gold is defined as 24 carat or 1000 fine. For dental alloys, the American Dental Association has classified the types of metal alloys based on noble metal content. In 2003, the Council for Scientific Affairs revised the classification to include titanium in a separate category because of its extensive usage and similar properties with noble metals (Table 2) [3,4].

E-mail address: dgivan@uab.edu

doi:10.1016/j.cden.2007.03.005

Table 1
Gold alloys commonly use carat and fineness classifications

Weight % gold	Carat	Fineness
100	24	1000
75	18	750
58	14	583
42	10	420

Precious alloys in dentistry are most commonly used in the form of castings. In 1907, Taggart [5] developed a process to cast metals using the lost-wax technique. The development of investment materials in the 1930s that matched the thermal expansion of the investment to that of the metal during the casting process significantly improved accuracy [6]. Gold alloys dominated the precious metal use in dentistry before the deregulation of gold prices on the open market in the late 1960s. During the next three decades, numerous alloys were introduced as lower cost substitutes for gold alloys. Current precious alloys most commonly use gold with various alloying elements, however, including palladium, platinum, silver, and copper, with combinations resulting in differing properties. Wataha [2] noted that the development of dental alloys have been influenced not only by economic factors but also by the need for improved physical and mechanical properties and concerns regarding corrosion and biocompatibility.

Casting alloys have been classified further by their yield strength and percent elongation in the American National Standards Institute/American Dental Association Specification No. 5 (Table 3) [7]. Casting alloys are designated as Type 1, 2, 3, or 4, with each alloy type recommended for specific usage. Type 3 castings are most commonly used in current dental practice. Types 1 and 2 offer limited resistance to oral forces, such as localized wear, but allow burnishability to mechanically improve the fit of a casting at the margin. Leinfelder [8] noted that type 3 castings also provide burnishability by heat softening after soaking for 10 to 15 minutes at 700°C followed by immediate quenching. The soft alloy can be burnished. After the burnishing procedure, the alloy is hardened by heating to 450°C for 30 minutes, cooling to 250 °C, and quenching to improve the its hardness and wear resistance.

Table 2
Revised American Dental Association classification of prosthodontic alloys

Class	Required noble content (%)	Required gold content (%)	Required titanium content (%)
High noble alloys	≥60	≥40	
Titanium and titanium alloys			≥85
Noble alloys	≥25		
Predominantly base metals	≥25		

Table 3
Classification of casting alloys: American National Standards Institute/American Dental Association specification number 5

Type	Designation	Minimum 0.2% yield strength	Minimum elongation (annealed) (%)	Recommended usage for castings
1	Low strength	80 MPa	18	Light stress (eg, inlays)
2	Medium strength	180 MPa	12	Moderate stress (eg, inlays and onlays)
3	High strength	240 MPa	12	High stress (eg, onlays, pontics, full crowns, short-span fixed partial dentures)
4	Extra high strength	300 MPa	10	High stress and thin cross-sections (eg, bars, thin veneer crowns, long-span fixed partial dentures, removable partial dentures)

Metallic elements in dental alloys

Metals commonly found in current dental casting alloys are shown in Table 4. Most precious dental alloys have two or three major elemental constituents with the addition of minor elements to influence specific properties, such as the melting range, grain formation, or resistance to corrosion. Gold is a major constituent of most precious dental alloys. Pure gold is the most ductile and malleable of all metals. It is resistant to corrosion and surface tarnish, which results in its noble status. These properties led to the use of gold as a direct filling material known as gold foil. Gold is yellow in color and is relatively insoluble in acids, with the exception of aqua regia, which is a combination of hydrochloric and nitric acids. Gold is dense and

Table 4
Metallic elements common in dental alloys

Element	Atomic mass	Melting point (°C)	Density (g/cm^2)	Comment
Gold (Au)	196.97	1064	19.32	Noble, precious
Palladium (Pd)	106.42	1554	12.02	Noble, precious
Platinum (Pt)	195.08	1772	21.45	Noble, precious
Iridum (Ir)	192.22	2410	22.65	Noble, precious
Ruthenium (Ru)	101.07	2310	12.48	Noble, precious
Rhodium (Rh)	102.91	1966	12.41	Noble, precious
Silver (Ag)	107.87	962	10.49	Base, precious
Copper (Cu)	63.55	1083	8.92	Base
Titanium (Ti)	47.87	1668	4.51	Light

provides excellent castability, and it has a relatively low melting point. It is highly conductive and has an elastic modulus and hardness similar to enamel, which results in a desirable wear coupled with teeth.

Palladium is a common constituent in many precious dental alloys. This metal was popularized as a low-cost substitute to gold; however, market fluctuations have dramatically increased the cost. Palladium is white in color and has a density approximately 60% that of gold. Palladium has a higher melting temperature than gold but may absorb hydrogen gas when heated, resulting in undesirable properties. Palladium has the unusual property of absorbing nearly 900 times its volume of hydrogen gas and is used in industry as a means of purifying hydrogen.

Platinum is a bright white metal characterized by high hardness and density. Platinum has a high melting point and resists oxidation at high temperatures. In foil form, it is used as a substrate for porcelain densification because it has a coefficient of thermal expansion similar to porcelain and a melting temperature higher than the porcelain sintering temperature. When alloyed with metals that have a lower melting temperature, such as gold, the resultant alloy may be compatible with ceramometal bonding. The high hardness imparts excellent resistance to wear and is a common constituent in precision prosthetic attachments. Although noble alloys generally have desirable biocompatibility [9,10], some reports have implicated platinum, along with palladium, in undesired biologic responses, such as hypersensitivity [11–13]. The evidence strongly supports the continued use of both metals in dentistry, however.

The remaining noble elements are less common metals in precious dental alloys but impart important properties to enhance the alloy's usefulness. Because of high melting temperatures, small amounts of iridium and ruthenium act as centers for nucleation and growth to reduce grain size when cooling after a casting procedure. Small grains are beneficial in improving mechanical properties of the alloy. These noble metals also are sometimes added to improve corrosion resistance to base metal dental alloys [14]. Rhodium and osmium have limited use in dentistry.

Silver is a common constituent in numerous dental alloys. Although some classify silver as precious or semi-precious because of financial value, it is not considered noble. Silver has a low melting temperature and readily uptakes oxygen, which makes it difficult to cast without porosity. Silver is reactive with sulfides, halides, and phosphates, which results in a surface tarnish. Silver forms solid solutions with gold and palladium, which improves the shortcomings of the pure metal for corrosion resistance and castability. Silver has been considered a whitening element for the color of dental alloys. Some silver alloys used for ceramometal bonding, especially with palladium, are considered to "green" porcelains, however, which results in a more yellowish appearance. At high temperature, silver diffuses into the porcelain, where it is reduced to form a colloidal metallic silver that results in a color change.

Numerous nonnoble elements are also common in precious dental alloys. Copper is present in many casting alloys, in which it forms solid solutions with gold and palladium to strengthen the alloy. Tin, indium, iron, zinc, and gallium are also common in small concentrations. Tin hardens platinum and palladium but may make the resultant alloy too brittle if used in too great a quantity. Zinc helps bind oxygen in the molten alloy but has minimal concentration in the final casting because of its low density and leaves most of the zinc in the casting "button." Because of its low melting point and high chemical activity, zinc is also a common element in many dental solders. Indium has been used as an oxygen scavenger and to "yellow" the alloy. Indium, tin, and gallium are used to enhance surface oxide formation necessary for ceramometal bonding.

Precious alloys for dental applications

Evaluation of precious alloys available to the dental market suggests a multitude of elemental combinations available for selection [15]. Examples of high noble and noble alloy compositions and properties are shown in Tables 5 and 6, respectively. If the alloy is intended for ceramometal bonding, the melting range must be higher than the porcelain firing temperatures to prevent distortion of the casting. The melting range describes the temperatures for the liquidus and solidus for a given composition. Constituents such as platinum and palladium are commonly used to counter the relatively low melting temperature of gold. Small amounts of high-temperature constituents, such as iridium, do not significantly influence the melting range of the alloy but affect the grain formation and resultant properties. The casting temperature is typically 50° to 100°C higher than the liquidus temperature and varies according to manufacturer recommendations. The

Table 5
Elemental constituents of common precious dental alloys

	%Au	%Pd	%Pt	%Ag	%Cu	%Other
High noble						
Au-Pt-Pd-Ag	78.00	12.00	6.00	1.20		1 Fe; <1 In, Sn, Ir
Au-Cu-Ag-Pd I	77.00	1.00		13.54	7.95	<1 Zn, Ir
Au-Cu-Ag-Pd II	60.00	3.75		26.70	8.80	<1 Zn, In, Ir
Au-Pt-Pd	86.00	1.95	10.00			2 In; <1 Ir
Au-Pd-Ag-In	40.00	37.40		15.00		6 In; 1.5 Ga; < 1 Ir
Noble						
Au-Cu-Ag-Pd III	46.00	6.00		39.50	7.49	1 Zn; <1 Ir
Pd-Cu-Ga		75.90			10.00	6.5 Ga; 7 In; <1 Ru
Ag-Pd		53.42		38.90		7 Sn; <1 Ga, Ru, Rh
Pd-Ga-Au	2.00	85.00				10 Ga; 1.1 In; <1 Ag, Ru
Pd-Ag-Au	6.00	75.00		6.50		6 In; 6 Ga; <1 Ru

Data courtesy of Jelenko Alloys, San Diego, CA; Ivoclar Vivaden, Amherst, NJ; Dentsply Ceramco, York, PA.

Table 6
Physical and mechanical properties of common precious dental alloys

	Melting range (°C)	Density (g/cc)	Heat treatment	Vicker's hardness (VHN)	Ultimate tensile strength (MPa)	Modulus of elasticity (GPa)	Percent elongation	Coefficient of thermal expansion (α × 10⁻⁶/°C)
High Noble								
Au-Pd-Pt-Ag	1170–1300	17.2	C	255	689	103.4	4%	14.3 @ 500 °C
Au-Cu-Ag-Pd I	920–980	15.8	A	145	434	82.7	44%	
Au-Cu-Ag-Pd II	900–990	14.2	B	165/245	455/689	–/96.5	45%/20%	
Au-Pt-Pd	1060–1230	18.7	C	190	586	82.7	6%	14.5 @ 500 °C
Au-Ag-Pd-In	1175–1280	13.0	C	265	586	124	17%	14.2 @ 500 °C
Noble								
Au-Cu-Ag-Pd III	900–1000	13.1	B	170/250	448/689	–/103.4	40%/20%	
Pd-Cu-Ga	1120–1270	10.5	C	365	1068	131	7%	13.8 @ 500 °C
Ag-Pd	1190–1300	10.9	C	220	689	115.8	25%	15.1 @ 500 °C
Pd-Ga-Au	1105–1330	10.9	C	285	717	131	25%	13.9 @ 500 °C
Pd-Ag-Au	1130–1340	11.0	C	250	827	131	35%	14.0 @ 500 °C

Heat treatments used before mechanical testing: A = quenched, B = quenched/hardened, C = porcelain firing cycle.
Data courtesy of Jelenko Alloys, San Diego, CA; Ivoclar Vivaden, Amherst, NJ; Dentsply Ceramco, York, PA.

investment materials must be compatible with the casting temperature used and the thermal expansion of the alloy.

The coefficient of thermal expansion is a measure of the change of material dimension as a function of temperature. During casting, the alloy contracts as it cools from the molten state. Investments are selected to match the expansion and contraction during the casting procedure. If the precious alloy is to be used for ceramometal bonding, then addition of platinum or palladium reduces the thermal expansion to be compatible with dental porcelain. Small amounts of oxide-forming constituents are included in the alloy for "degassing," which refers to a controlled heat treatment that forms a surface oxide layer on the alloy. The bond between the veneering porcelain is considered to be a combination of mechanical retention, Van der Waals interactions, compressive bonding, and chemical bonding with the oxide layer [16,17]. The chemical bond is considered to be the most significant contribution for the strength of the bond. The alloy should have a slightly greater coefficient of thermal expansion than the ceramic, however, in which during cooling the alloy surface contracts more than the ceramic and results in a compressive stress within the ceramic and a tensile stress in the metal. Ceramics are generally weak in tension but strong under compression because of a tendency to close initial crack flaws within the ceramic, which inhibits crack propagation and failure of the ceramometal bond. Precious alloys used for ceramometal bonding may have coefficients of thermal expansion influenced by minor constituents in the alloy and have a typical range of 13.5 to 14.5 $\times$ 10^{-6}/°C. Porcelains frequently have a range slightly less: 13 to 14 $\times$ 10^{-6}/°C.

The composition of precious alloys influences other physical and mechanical properties. Density of an alloy is related to the proportion of the density from each constituent. Because low-density constituents, such as silver and palladium, are used in greater concentrations to reduce the amount of gold, the overall density of the alloy is decreased, which reduces castability with the centrifugal casting method [18]. The hardness of the alloy is similarly affected by the alloy composition. The hardness, which is the resistance to plastic deformation upon indentation, gives an indication of the susceptibility to surface abrasion, ease of finishing and polishing, and an estimation of the counter-surface wear potential against enamel. Enamel has a Vickers hardness of approximately 294 VHN [19]. Most precious alloys have a hardness less than enamel and are considered to be favorable wear couples in which the alloy is abraded rather than tooth structure. Elongation, which gives a measure of ductility, burnishability, and flexibility, is also affected by the alloy composition (Table 6). Finally, the elemental constituents of precious alloys have an impact on biocompatibility. In general, noble and high noble alloys have excellent passivity, which results in a good resistance to intraoral corrosion. Allergenic potential is considered to be a low risk, although some concerns have been raised regarding the use of platinum and palladium.

High noble alloys can be considered in three groups: Au-Pt, Au-Pd, and Au-Ag-Cu alloys (refer to Table 4 for elemental symbols). Au-Pt alloys are used for full-metal and ceramometal applications. This alloy type was formulated to include platinum as a palladium substitute for economic reasons [20]. Platinum has a high melting temperature and adds resistance to sagging distortion during porcelain firing. The resultant alloy is white and may be strengthened by iron, zinc, or silver. Traces of iron present in some formulations result in the formation of an intermetallic phase to strengthen the alloy. Other formulations may include zinc, which forms a dispersed phase, or silver, which is soluble with gold for solid solution strengthening. Indium and tin readily form a surface oxide for porcelain bonding, which diffuses to the surface in high concentration during the porcelain firing cycles [21].

Au-Pd alloys are a popular high noble dental casting alloy despite the high cost. This white alloy may include oxide formers, such as indium and iridium, and is a common choice for ceramometal restorations. Some formulations include silver for solid solution hardening. As a class of alloys, Au-Pd alloys have higher strength, modulus, and hardness over the gold-platinum alloys. A high palladium content reduces the density of the alloy, however, and affects the force of the alloy as it enters the investment during casting. Despite the lower density, this alloy type is considered relatively easy to cast [18].

Au-Ag-Cu high noble alloys have been used for many years for full-metal applications. The temperature of the solidus is too low for ceramometal bonding. Copper, like silver, also may affect the color of the porcelain and impart a reddish-brown appearance. The alloy is yellow in color and easily cast and soldered. Silver is a common constituent of the alloys, and copper and silver are miscible in gold, which results in a single phase alloy. Craig and Powers [18] further categorized copper-containing high noble alloys by the gold content. Lower gold alloys have a much higher silver content, which can affect casting density of the alloy and decrease the corrosion resistance. Heat treatments are used to harden or soften this high noble alloy by solution hardening and ordered hardening. For most type 3 and type 4 casting alloys, this hardening involves copper. Types 1 and 2 typically do not contain enough copper to be hardened by this mechanism and are not recommended for full crowns or fixed partial dentures.

The noble alloys may be considered in three groups: Au-Ag-Pd, low-gold alloys, including such as Pd-Ag and Pd-Ga, and no-gold alloys, such as Pd-Cu-Ga. The Au-Ag-Pd alloys are characterized as having less than 50% gold and a high silver content. This alloy was developed as a lower cost alternative when the price of gold dramatically increased in the early 1980s. Au-Ag-Pd noble alloys are usually single phase, which may be hardened by solid solution strengthening. Copper is a common element in this alloy type and is similar to the high noble alloy in structure and properties. In some formulations, the amount of palladium and copper is significantly increased while the gold content is decreased, which results in a sagging resistance to be less than the other noble alloys. Overall, the properties of this alloy group are generally good with acceptable strength and hardness but only moderate ductility [1]. Corrosion resistance may worsen as the silver and copper concentration increases [22].

Pd-Ag silver alloys are another alternative alloy developed as a gold substitute. This alloy type was associated with problems of "greening" porcelain caused by the reduction of silver. Pd-Ga alloys became popular to avoid the problems associated with silver. Indium, ruthenium, and tin are frequently added for the dual purpose of strengthening the alloy and forming a surface oxide for porcelain bonding. Gallium reduces the liquidus temperature, which was increased by the palladium content, improves porcelain bonding, and enhances the strength [23]. A fine precipitate has been shown in radiographic diffraction studies to develop at the grain boundaries, which further increases hardness [24]. Anusavice [25] noted that subsurface oxides may form with Pd-Ga alloys. Although it has not been shown to be detrimental to performance, it is less than ideal because the interface may become brittle. The surface of Pd-Ga alloys forms nodules to create an irregular surface to retain porcelain by mechanical rather than chemical mechanisms.

Some precious dental alloy formations do not include any gold, such as Pd-Cu-Ga alloys. This low-cost alternative alloy has favorable hardness similar to tooth structure and excellent casting accuracy. Care should be taken in casting because contamination from the crucible or the investment has been problematic [21]. A high hardness Pd_2Ga_5 precipitate forms at the grain boundaries in some formulations, which significantly increases hardness. Concerns have been raised regarding the biocompatibility of high-palladium alloys. Extensive research has been reviewed to support the safety and efficacy of this alloy group [26].

Wrought alloys

Alloys that undergo cold working treatments, such as flattening in a rolling mill or drawing to form a wire, are work hardened by mechanical compression and reshaping of the grains. These alloys are known as "wrought alloys" and are used for various purposes in dentistry, including precision attachments, backings of denture teeth, and removable partial denture clasps [18]. Nearly all wrought dental alloys are precious alloys, being either high noble or noble. Gold-based wrought alloys commonly have approximately 60% Au and may be alloyed with Ag, Cu, Pd, and Pt. Formulations available without gold, such as a Pd-Ag-Cu alloy. Care must be taken when heating the alloy during soldering or during "cast to" procedures to avoid recrystallization of the alloy removing the cold-worked grain structure. Advantages of wrought alloys include increased toughness and enhanced elongation, which are beneficial for applications that require adjustment by plastic deformation or flexibility.

Soldering and brazing

Metals can be joined by three similar processes: welding, brazing, and soldering [27]. Welding is a fusion of two metals to join the pieces by a localized heating above the liquidus. A filler metal is sometimes used but is not necessary. Welds in dentistry are often accomplished with a laser. The area adjacent to the fused metal is known as the "heat affected zone," in which partial recrystallization of the alloy is probable. A decrease in hardness is noted when measured across a welded joint as a result of recrystallization. Minimizing the duration and area of heating reduces the heat affected zone.

Brazing and soldering join metals at a temperature below the solidus using a third low-melting-point metal. Traditionally, brazing occurs at a temperature of more than 1000°F (538 °C), whereas soldering occurs at a lesser temperature. Much of the soldering in dentistry is more accurately described as brazing. The filler alloy is referred to as a "solder" and is typically gold-based alloy for good compatibility with the alloys to be joined. Craig and Powers [18] described the ideal qualities of a solder, which should include ease of flow at low temperatures, free flow in the melt state, strength and color similar to pieces to be joined, and resistance to tarnish, corrosion, and pitting upon heating. Most precious alloy dental solders are an Au-Ag-Cu alloy with additions of Sn and Zn. Fusion temperatures range from approximately 700° to 850°C but must remain below the temperature of the alloy being soldered. The strength of the solder alloy is enhanced by slower cooling for order hardening. The strength of the joint is often more affected by soldering technique and influenced by the distance between pieces, cross-section of the solder joint, and proper use of heat, flux, and investment. For example, overheating the solder alloy well above the liquidus can preferentially separate zinc and tin from the melt and result in pitting.

Summary

Precious alloys are an important material group in dentistry because of their ease of use, excellent compatibility, favorable mechanical and physical properties, and application in ceramometal bonding. Although new precious alloys have been introduced in the past decades, frequently because of economic pressure, gold-based alloys remain a popular choice. Wataha [2] suggested that alloys should be chosen based on an understanding of the alloy system, selection of proven alloys from quality manufacturers, and consideration of the requirements of a given clinical situation.

References

[1] O'Brien WJ. Dental materials and their selection. 3rd edition. Chicago: Quintessence Publishing Co., Inc.; 2002.

[2] Wataha JC. Alloys for prosthodontic restorations. J Prosthet Dent 2002;87(4):351–63.

[3] ADA Council on Scientific Affairs. Titanium applications in dentistry. J Am Dent Assoc 2003;134(3):347–9.

[4] ADA Council on Scientific Affairs Positions & Statements. Revised classification system for alloys for fixed prosthodontics. Available at: http://www.ada.org/prof/resources/positions/ statements/prosthodontics.asp. Accessed September 12, 2006.

[5] Taggart WH. A new and accurate method of making gold inlays. The Dental Cosmos 1907; 49:1117–21.

[6] Scheu CH. Controlled hygroscopic expansion of investment to compensate for shrinkage in inlay casting. J Am Dent Assoc 1935;22:452–5.

[7] ANSI/ADA. Specification No. 5: dental casting alloys. Chicago: American Dental Association; 1997.

[8] Leinfelder KF. An evaluation of casting alloys used for restorative procedures. J Am Dent Assoc 1997;128(1):37–45.

[9] Al-Hiyasat AS, Darmani H, Bashabsheh OM. Cytotoxicity of dental casting alloys after conditioning in distilled water. Int J Prosthodont 2003;16(6):597–601.

[10] Grill V, Sandrucci MA, Di Lenarda R, et al. In vitro evaluation of the biocompatibility of dental alloys: fibronectin expression patterns and relationships to cellular proliferation rates. Quintessence Int 2000;31(10):741–7.

[11] Schierl R. Urinary platinum levels associated with dental gold alloys. Arch Environ Health 2001;56(3):283–6.

[12] Mizoguchi S, Setoyama M, Kanzaki T. Linear lichen planus in the region of the mandibular nerve caused by an allergy to palladium in dental metals. Dermatology 1998;196(2):268–70.

[13] Koch P, Baum HP. Contact stomatitis due to palladium and platinum in dental alloys. Contact Dermatitis 1996;34(4):253–7.

[14] Reclaru L, Luthy H, Eschler P-Y, et al. Corrosion behaviour of cobalt-chromium dental alloys doped with precious metals. Biomaterials 2005;26(21):4358–65.

[15] Moffa JP. Alternative dental casting alloys. Dent Clin North Am 1983;27(4):733–46.

[16] McLean JW, Hughes TH. The reinforcement of dental porcelain with ceramic oxides. Br Dent J 1965;119:251–67.

[17] Leinfelder KF, Lemons JE. Clinical restorative materials and techniques. Philadelphia: Lea & Febiger; 1988.

[18] Craig RG, Powers JM. Restorative dental materials. St. Louis (MO): Mosby; 2002.

[19] Forss H, Seppa L, Lappalainen R. In vitro abrasion resistance and hardness of glass-ionomer cements. Dent Mater 1991;7:36–9.

[20] Wataha JC, Messer RL. Casting alloys. Dent Clin North Am 2004;48(2):499–512.

[21] Brantley WA, Laub LW. Metal selection. In: Rosenstiel SF, Land MF, Fujimoto J, editors. Contemporary fixed prosthodontics. 4th edition. St. Louis (MO): Elsevier; 2006. p. 599–609.

[22] Wataha JC, Lockwood PE. Release of elements from dental casting alloys into cell-culture medium over 10 months. Dent Mater 1998;14(2):158–63.

[23] Wu Q, Brantley WA, Mitchell JC, et al. Heat-treatment behavior of high-pallidium dental alloys. Cells Mater 1997;7:161–74.

[24] Brantley WA, Cai Z, Foreman DW, et al. X-ray diffraction studies of as-cast high-palladium alloys. Dent Mater 1995;11(3):154–60.

[25] Anusavice KJ. Phillip's science of dental materials. 10th edition. Philadelphia: W.B. Saunders; 1996.

[26] Wataha JC, Hanks CT. Biological effects of palladium and risk of using palladium in dental casting alloys. J Oral Rehabil 1996;23(5):309–20.

[27] Flinn RA, Trojan PK. Engineering materials and their applications. Boston: Houghton Mifflin Company; 1990.

ELSEVIER
SAUNDERS

Dent Clin N Am 51 (2007) 603–627

THE DENTAL
CLINICS
OF NORTH AMERICA

Base Metal Alloys Used for Dental Restorations and Implants

Michael Roach, MS

Department of Biomedical Materials Research, University of Mississippi Medical Center
School of Dentistry, 2500 North State Street, Jackson, MS 39216, USA

The history of dental restorations and implants dates back to the ancient Egyptians, who used sea shells on corpses for burial, and the Etruscans, who used bone and bands of gold wire to replace missing teeth [1]. The modern era of dental restorations began just after the turn of the 20th century with the use of a number of precious metals, as well as some attempts to use zinc, steel, copper, and even brass [1,2]. The success of some of these materials as well as fluctuations in the cost and availability of gold, which exploded to nearly $900 an ounce in 1980, have been credited with driving dentistry toward the development and use of alternative metal alloys [2–5]. During the 20th century, the efforts of numerous researchers have lead to the development of new alloys that are not only less expensive than gold, but have properties more suitable for specific applications. Many of the modern alloy systems do not include precious metals as previously used in dentistry. Because the primary alloying elements for these alloys do not include precious metals, they are referred to as base metal alloys. In this article, five base metals alloy systems used in dentistry—stainless steels, nickel-chrome alloys, cobalt-chromium alloys, titanium alloys, and super-elastic nickel-titanium alloys—are described in the order of their introduction into the field.

Stainless steel alloys

Stainless steels have been successfully used in orthopedics and dentistry for almost a full century. Sherman [6] introduced vanadium surgical steel in 1912, when he found that it possessed elasticity and ductility not found in other steels; however, the vanadium steel had poor biocompatibility. In

E-mail address: mroach@sod.umsmed.edu

1926, the 18-8—18% chromium (Cr)-8% nickel (Ni)—austenitic stainless steel was introduced because it was stronger and more corrosion-resistant in saline environments. Later that same year, Strauss [7] patented a variation of this 18-8 steel that added 2% to 4% molybdenum (Mo) and made it even more resistant in acidic and chloride environments. The carbon content of this 18Cr-8Ni-Mo alloy was later lowered to 0.08%, and the alloy became known as 316 stainless steel. As is seen from the history of the development of austenitic stainless steel, the composition is based upon iron with the addition of chromium, nickel, and often molybdenum as the primary alloying elements. Chromium and molybdenum are added for corrosion resistance and significant amounts of nickel are added to stabilize the austenitic structure. Additional common alloying elements include silicon, manganese, niobium, titanium, and carbon. Although austenitic steels are not hardenable by heat treatments, the large amount of ductility allows them to undergo substantial cold working before fracture [8]. The major austenitic stainless steels used in dentistry today are still the same 18-8 (302 and 304) and 316 alloy.

Since its introduction in the form of hand-drawn archwire around 1929, 18-8 stainless steel has been extensively used in dentistry [9]. During the 1960s, stainless steel orthodontic wires were overtaking gold because of the higher stiffness, and the smaller, more esthetic, size of the restoration [2]. Because of their low costs, good mechanical properties, and adequate corrosion resistance in the oral environment, austenitic stainless steels are commonly used today for orthodontic wire and appliances, temporary crowns, magnetic connectors and clips, and dental implants [9–11].

As shown in Table 1 [12–23], the 18-8 stainless steel orthodontic archwires are considerably stronger than the cobalt-chromium nickel (Co-Cr-Ni), titanium-molybdenum (Ti-Mo), and nickel-titanium (Ni-Ti) wires. The manufacturing process of stainless steel wires cold-works the material, which reduces its ductility. A recovery heat treatment process between 400°C and 500°C will relieve such residual stresses in the material from manufacturing and thus improve its elastic properties [8]. Several additional mechanical property terms used in classifying orthodontic wire are outside of those normally described in material property characterization. Formability has been defined as the ability to bend the wire into the configuration desired by the clinician [9]; 18-8 stainless steel wires have been shown to have excellent formability [24]. Stiffness is proportional to the elastic modulus, and is a measure of the force applied by the restoration to the teeth [9]. As shown in Table 1, the elastic modulus of stainless steel is approximately twice that of gold, but lower than the Co-Cr-Ni wires, and therefore stainless steel wires have a stiffness value in between the gold and Co-Cr-Ni wires. Resiliency reflects the work ability of the wire acting as a spring [5,25]. Stainless steel wires have a favorable resiliency compared with gold wires, and have been shown to be able to do the work needed clinically to move teeth [5]. Flexibility or springback is defined as the materials maximum elastic deflection, and is the ratio of the yield strength over the modulus of elasticity [9,25]. The springback of stainless steel wires has been shown to be slightly higher than that of gold wires, but lower than most Ti-Mo and Ni-Ti wires [9,24]. Finally, the joinability of a wire is the ability to weld or solder to attachments. Soldering of the stainless steel wires is possible, but can be somewhat difficult [24].

In general, the 18-8 stainless steel orthodontic wires have shown at least adequate corrosion resistance in the oral environment. Kim and Johnson [26] performed a potentiodynamic comparative study of 18-8 stainless steel, Ti-Mo, and Ni-Ti orthodontic wires in a 0.9% sodium chloride (NaCl) solution, and recorded an oxide film breakdown potential (E_{br}) of 400 mV for the stainless steel. This E_{br} value was inside the range of those reported for Ni-Ti, but significantly less than those for the Ti-Mo wire. The stainless steel wire corroded readily in the saline solution and revealed more surface pitting when compared with the Ni-Ti wires, indicating that the stainless steel is more susceptible to corrosion; however, Sarkar and colleagues [27] performed a similar cyclic polarization study of the common types of orthodontic wires in a 1% NaCl solution and found no oxide breakdown in the stainless steel orthodontic wire, whereas the Ni-Ti wire showed oxide layer breakdown and extensive pitting corrosion. In this study, the potentials were only driven to +300 millivolts (mV) versus standard calomel electrode (SCE), and the Ni-Ti wire still experienced oxide breakdown at a potential slightly over +100 mV versus SCE. In addition, Lin and colleagues [28] showed that the brand of commercially available 18-8 stainless steel orthodontic bracket, and thus the processing techniques, showed more of an effect on the corrosion resistance of the appliance than differences in initial surface roughness or manufacturing defects. Shin and colleagues [29] found similar results in an immersion study on stainless steel orthodontic archwires, stress relieved at 500°C, in artificial saliva. This study concluded that uniform surface corrosion was detected on the heat-treated arch wires after a 12-week immersion in artificial saliva. Crevice corrosion was also observed between the brackets and banding material. The corrosion resistance of stainless steels with higher carbon contents may be decreased during heat treatments between 400°C and 900°C, through the formation of chromium-iron carbides at the grain boundaries. These chromium-iron carbides result in a localized chromium depletion in the oxide layer, thus creating intergranular corrosion [8]. Therefore, the corrosion shown by Shin and colleagues [29] may have been caused by the formation of chromium-iron carbides at the grain boundaries. Kerosuo and colleagues [30] found significantly greater releases of nickel from a fixed stainless steel orthodontic appliance under dynamic conditions simulating more realistic in vivo applications, as compared with static dissolution. Chromium release was also detected from this appliance, but was not significantly different comparing static and dynamic dissolution conditions [30]. Nonetheless, Staffolani and colleagues [31] determined daily Ni and Cr release levels from orthodontic appliances in acid solutions to be well below the levels ingested in the daily diet.

Table 1
Physical and mechanical properties of dental metal materials

Alloy	Condition	Tensile strength (MPa)	Yield strength (MPa)	Elastic modulus (GPa)	Elongation (%)	Density (g/cm^3)
Stainless steel						
18-8 wire [12,24,25,53,98]	As received	2035–2849	965–1680	134–200	2–3.2	8
	Stress relieved	2160	1034–1950	134–200	—	8
316 wire [35]	As received	2275–2351	1955–2070	185–191	—	—
316L [13,14,41,108]	Annealed	550–600	220–331	190–200	50–55	7.95
	Cold-worked	896–1014	790–827	167–200	20–25	7.9–7.95
108 [41,50]	Annealed	931	586	188	52	7.63
	Cold-worked	1344	1179	188	35	7.63
Nickel-Chromium						
Ni-Cr-Be [15,54]	Casting	778–1355	325–838	165–210	3–23.9	7.9–8.1
Ni-Cr [15,54]	Casting	539–919	180–858	141–248	<1–32.6	7.9–8.7
Cobalt-Chromium						
Co-Cr-Mo [16,53,54,108,119]	Casting	655–889	390–644	155–240	1.5–10	8.5
Co-Ni-Cr-Mo [13,14,16,99]	Wrought/annealed	795–1007	240–655	232	50–70	9.2
Co-Cr-Ni [8]	Casting	685	470	198	8.0	7.5–8.5
Co-Cr-Ni wire [17,18,24,98]	As received	—	827–1241	146–198	—	7.5–8.5
	Stress relieved	—	1103–1378	179–204	8.0	7.5–8.5
Titanium						
CP Ti [53,114]	Casting	240–550	170–480	96–114	7.9–20	4.4–4.5
CP Ti—grade 1 [16,19,108]	Annealed	240	170	100–103	24	4.51

Material	Condition					
CP Ti—grade 2 [16,35,108]	Annealed	345	275	100–103	20	4.51
CP Ti—grade 3 [16,19,108]	Annealed	450	380	100–103	18	4.51
CP Ti—grade 4 [16,19,108]	Annealed	550	485	100–104	15	4.51
CP Ti—grade 4 [13,122]	Cold-worked	760–888	485–725	110	—	4.51
Ti-6Al-4V ELI [13,14,16,19,108,122]	Annealed	860–1076	520–896	110–116	10–15	4.43–4.5
Ti-6Al-4V [8,14,114,119]	Casting	877–930	830–870	113–137	2.1–12	—
Ti-6Al-7Nb [19,122]	Annealed	978–1024	913	105	—	4.52
Ti-15Mo [20,122]	Annealed/aged	874	544	78	—	4.96
TMA wire [21,98]	As drawn	—	621–1172	60–69.6	—	—
	Heat-treated/aged	—	1220–1390	92.4–95.1	—	—
Nickel-Titanium			—	—	—	—
Ni-Ti wire-A [22,24,127]		527–1380	230–379	120	13–40	6.45
Ni-Ti wire-M [98,127]		—	207–552	32–50	—	—
Other			—	—	—	—
Pure gold [108]		130	20	90	45	19.3
Type III and IV		—	—	—	—	—
Gold casting [8,108]		—	207–434	90	10–39	11.3–15.5
Cortical bone [23,108]		100–200	130	10–20	1–3	0.7 (dry)
Cancellous bone [23]		10–20	—	0.2–0.5	5–7	—

Abbreviations: ELI, extra low interstitial; GPa, gigapascal; MPa, megapascal.

In addition to orthodontic wire applications, 18-8 stainless steels have also been used for adolescent and temporary adult preformed metal crowns for more than 50 years [32]. In addition to low costs, stainless steel crowns offer good corrosion resistance, ductility, and the ability to work-harden during the crimping process. Some clinicians have suggested these pre-formed stainless crowns to be easier to place in certain difficult patients, such as a crying child, when compared with amalgams [32]; however, other practitioners suggest that these restorations are too time-consuming to fit, inappropriate for many applications, difficult to manipulate, and not aes-thetically pleasing in the oral cavity [33].

Some manufacturers have elected to use a more corrosion-resistant 316 steel in place of the more prevalent 302/304 stainless steel used in orthodon-tics. Peterson recommended the 316 alloy shortly after WWII as the steel with the best combination of properties for bone plates and screws used for fracture fixation treatments by the Army [34]. Some time after that, it was introduced as a new orthodontic wire in dentistry. The addition of 2% to 4% Mo to 316 gave this new orthodontic wire superior corrosion resistance in addition to its superior elastic properties, compared with 18-8 steels [35]. Further studies on orthodontic brackets and molar bands have suggested reduced staining of the enamel and metal ion release in 316 compared with 18-8 orthodontic brackets and bands [31,36].

During the 1950s, the carbon content of 316 was lowered from 0.08% to 0.03%, and an 'L" (low carbon) was added to the designation (316L). In the 1960s and 1970s, implant retrieval studies and research suggested the need to make further changes in the composition requirements of implant- qual-ity 316L stainless steel (American Society of Testing Materials [ASTM] F138 [37]) by adjusting the limits of Ni, Cr, and Mo [38]. The ASTM F138 standard uses a compositional pitting resistance equivalent (PRE) function to insure that the Cr and Mo levels are adequate to control pitting corrosion. The tighter restrictions on Cr and Mo levels under ASTM F138 make 316L more corrosion-resistant than the 18-8 and 316 steels commonly used in dentistry. This additional corrosion resistance translates to lower metal ion release levels into the surrounding tissues, and thus less chance of an inflammatory reaction by the patient and less device loosening over time [39,40]. Several studies have characterized the mechanical [41], tor-sional [42], notched sensitivity [41], corrosion [43], stress corrosion cracking [41], and smooth and notched corrosion fatigue properties [38,44] of implant quality 316L, and compared them with other austenitic stainless steels used for implants. Because most implant failures in vivo are caused by fatigue, the corrosion fatigue performance of these materials in saline environments at physiological temperatures is of particular interest. Showing a lower smooth sample fatigue strength compared with other austenitic steels used in orthopedics, 316L demonstrated the lowest fatigue notch sensitivity of the group. Therefore, the presence of a defect or scratch in the device should not substantially accelerate the failure of a 316L appliance or implant in vivo.

Nickel is the most hypersensitive metal, and is a major component of most austenitic stainless steels. Although 10% to 20% of the population is hypersensitive to nickel, relatively few of these sensitive individuals have experienced metal sensitivity reactions caused by implants [45,46]. Nevertheless, the potential accumulation of nickel from the release over the lifetime of a restoration or implant remains a concern for patient hypersensitivity reactions. In part as a response to concerns over such sensitivity reactions, low-nickel ($\leq 0.05\%$) austenitic stainless steels have recently been developed, providing a "nickel-free" alternative and presenting some interesting mechanical and corrosion properties. Instead of adding nickel, these alloys use a high nitrogen content ($>0.90\%$) to stabilize the austenitic microstructure. This high nitrogen content also strengthens the alloy and contributes to its corrosion resistance [47–49]. Corrosion studies on one such alloy, BioDur108 (108) (Carpenter Technology, Wyomissing, Pennsylvania), in the laboratories of the author's institution [43] revealed a large passive range, with an E_{br} value that is far superior to 316L, as shown in Fig. 1. In the same austenitic steel studies mentioned above, 30% cold-worked 108 showed the highest smooth and notched sample fatigue strengths. In addition, this nitrogen-strengthened austenitic steel retained substantial ductility after 30% cold working (see Table 1). The strength of annealed 108 is similar to cold-worked 316L, and the ductility of 108 is far superior (see Table 1). Fatigue studies on 108 in the annealed condition are currently under way in the author's institution's laboratories. The combination of superior ductility, fatigue strengths, and low levels of nickel ($<0.05\%$) in the composition make this alloy worth consideration for future dental use [50].

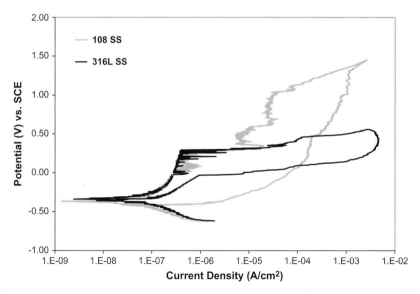

Fig. 1. Representative potentiodynamic curves of stainless steels in Ringer's solution at 37°C.

Nickel-chromium alloys

Because of the lower cost of nickel compared with gold, starting in the 1930s, Ni-Cr castings such as Lunorium (Salabes Research Laboratories, Inc., Baltimore, Maryland) [5], Ticonium (Albany, New York) [51], and those meeting the composition requirements under the Touceda [52] patent were introduced for crowns, bridges, and partial denture frameworks. In addition to the financial benefits, the Ni-Cr alloys have superior properties for use in porcelain-fused-to-metal (PFM) applications. These superior properties include a higher hardness values and substantially higher modulus of elasticity when compared with gold, as shown in Table 1. This increase in the modulus of elasticity allows the cross-sectional thickness of the restoration to be decreased, and allows more space for the porcelain veneer, while still providing the appropriate strengths [3,53,54]. Also, the thermal coefficients of expansion of the Ni-Cr alloys is closer to the porcelain veneers, which helps prevent cracking during heating and cooling cycles encountered by the restoration [55].

Ni-Cr alloys are generally divided into groupings based on the chromium, molybdenum, and beryllium (Be) content in the bulk composition. A number of researchers have separated the alloys into two or three compositional groupings with some variations in the exact criteria. A combination of the divisional criteria of some of these researchers yields three alloy classes: (1) Ni High-Cr (16%–27% Cr) High-Mo (>6% Mo), (2) Ni-Cr, and (3) Ni-Cr-Be (beryllium added) alloys [54,56–61]. Be is added to enhance castability by lowering the melting range of the alloy and also as a grain refiner [3,53]. O'Connor and colleagues [62] found Ni-Cr-Be alloys to cast almost twice the number of segments as the next alloy grouping, in a large-scale dental alloy casting study that included Ni-Cr-Be, Ni-Cr, and Co-Cr as well as noble and precious alloys systems. In addition, the same study showed that the beryllium-containing Ni-Cr alloys produced better porcelain-metal bonds compared with the Ni-Cr alloys without beryllium. Molybdenum, titanium, and manganese additions all increase corrosion resistance [63,64]. Molybdenum is also added to decrease the thermal expansion coefficient [53]. Aluminum additions increase strength and hardness [4,53]. In partial denture frameworks, carbon is added for enhanced yield strength and hardness, but it reduces ductility [53,63]. The numerous alloying elements available in the Ni-Cr alloys present a wide range of microstructures with solid solution matrixes and intermetallic compounds. The heterogeneous surfaces and oxide layers contribute to a wide range of corrosion resistance, because of preferential ion release from certain areas on the surface, which may lead to internal galvanic coupling.

The wide range of corrosion response in Ni-Cr dental alloys allows the three compositional groupings mentioned earlier to also be separated by their corrosion resistance to acidic or chloride-containing solutions. Fig. 2 provides representative cyclic polarization scans from unpublished research data comparing the three classes of Ni-Cr alloys in a lactic acid-based

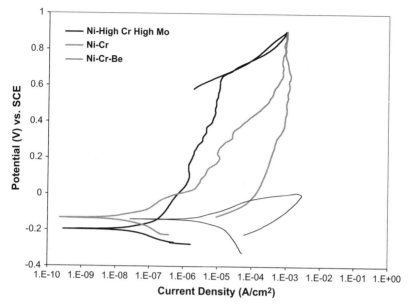

Fig. 2. Representative potentiodynamic curves of three Ni-Cr dental casting alloys in artificial saliva at 37°C.

artificial saliva solution at pH 4.6. The representative Ni High-Cr High-Mo alloy provided the lowest corrosion rate, as represented by the low corrosion current density (I_{corr}) value, and the highest breakdown or pitting potential (E_{br}) of the three alloy classes, which translates to a lower amount of metal ion release, and thus less chance of an allergic reaction by the patient. In cyclic polarization tests, the area of the hysteresis between the forward and reverse voltage scans is indicative of the amount of pitting corrosion taking place. Pitting corrosion changes the area and possibly the composition of the surface and oxide layers, and thus changes the alloy response, which creates an area mismatch between the forward and reverse scans. The Ni High-Cr High-Mo alloy revealed no hysteresis between the forward and reverse scans, indicating a lack of pitting corrosion. The Ni-Cr alloy showed a similar corrosion rate, but a substantially lower E_{br} value, and a hysteresis between the forward and reverse scans, suggesting a less stable oxide and lower pitting resistance. Finally, the Ni-Cr-Be alloy revealed significantly higher I_{corr} values, even lower E_{br} values, and a large hysteresis, indicating a substantially significant increase in pitting corrosion rate and thus metal ion release into the surrounding tissues, compared with the other Ni-Cr alloys. Several studies have shown that the release of metal ions from all classes of Ni-Cr casting alloys is not proportional with the bulk alloy composition [60,65–67]. Metal ion release from Ni-Cr alloys is normally mostly nickel, but the alloying element release can vary substantially because of selective leaching. Acidic environments can substantially increase the amount of nickel released. Wataha and colleagues [68] reported more nickel release in 30 minutes in an acid environment than a full year in a neutral environment. In Ni-Cr-Be alloys, Be ions are released at an accelerated rate, because of the Ni-Be eutectic phase that is selectively attacked on the surface of the alloy. Bumgardner and Lucas [67] found that Be ions were released initially at four to six times the bulk Ni-Cr-Be alloy composition in a cell culture dissolution study in 5% fetal bovine serum. Tai and colleagues [69], also studying a Ni-Cr-Be alloy system, concluded that occlusal wear may further increase metal ion release of nickel and beryllium to two or three times the levels from dissolution alone.

It should also be noted that the mechanical and corrosion properties of these alloys may be significantly affected by the heat treatments used during the PFM firing cycle. Winkler and colleagues [70] and Marinello and colleagues [71] reported decreases in hardness, and Morris [72] found a significant reduction in strength on Ni-based alloys, after the PFM firing cycle. Roach and colleagues [61] showed a substantial increase in corrosion rates for the Ni High-Cr High-Mo class and some of the Ni-Cr alloy class as a result of heat treatments used in porcelain firing, whereas Ni-Cr-Be alloys were not significantly affected. An important side note from this study was that the oxide breakdown potentials of the alloys were not significantly affected by the PFM firing processes, which agreed with studies by De Micheli [73] and Meyer [64].

Because between 10% and 20% for the population is hypersensitive to nickel, the release of metal ions from Ni-based restorations into the surrounding tissues is a primary concern [46,60,66,67]. In general, women also demonstrate a higher sensitivity to nickel than men, in part because of sensitization caused by jewelry containing nickel [74,75]. Despite the hypersensitivity of some patients to nickel, Jones and colleagues [76] concluded that a history of nickel allergy does not necessarily prevent a patient from successfully wearing a nickel-containing prosthesis.

Cobalt-chromium alloys

Cast cobalt-chromium materials

In 1907 Haynes patented cobalt-chromium (Co-Cr) stellite alloys, and later added tungsten and molybdenum to increase hardness, strength and abrasion resistance [5,77]. It took until 1929 for Co-Cr alloys to be used in dental appliances, when Erdle and Prange of Austenal laboratories (York, Pennsylvania) developed Co-Cr-W (tungsten) and Co-Cr-Mo casting alloys [5,78–80]. The Co-Cr-Mo alloy was later given the trade name Vitallium in 1932. In the mid to late 1930s, Venable and Stuck [81,82] performed studies on a series of alloys available at the time, including this new Co-Cr-Mo alloy, to determine the effects of electrolysis on bone and surrounding tissues.

They found the Vitallium to have superior resistance to bodily fluids and no effect on the surrounding tissues or bone. In 1939, Dr. Strock implanted "venable screws" of this Co-Cr-Mo alloy into humans, resulting in the first-ever bone growth around a metallic implant, even though these implants would soon fail. Over the next couple of decades, the use of the Co-Cr alloys for partial denture restorations was continuing to increase, and by 1950 it was estimated that five times as many partial dentures were made of Co-Cr alloys than were made of gold [78].

Chromium is a key component of these alloys because of its tarnish and corrosion resistance; however, adding more than 30% chromium makes this alloy difficult to cast and can result in a brittle sigma phase, so dental casting alloys should not contain more than 29% [53,83]. Cobalt increases the elastic modulus and strength to higher levels than nickel [4,53]. Molybdenum is added to lower the thermal expansion coefficient and adds to the corrosion resistance [53]. Tungsten increases corrosion resistance and reduces Cr-depleted intermetallic areas [4]. Nickel increases ductility while lowering the hardness of the alloy [78,84]. Silicon, manganese, carbon, and iron are additional alloying elements in cobalt-based alloys [11]. Many of these alloying elements react with carbon to form carbides, and thus change the properties of the Co-Cr alloys [53]. With the large number of alloying elements, the Co-Cr alloys exhibit a nonhomogeneous microstructure similar to that of the Ni-Cr base alloys. The microstructure is made up of a solid-solution austenitic matrix with intermetallic compounds [53]. This alloy system presents hardness values, strengths, and modulus values in similar ranges to those of the Ni-Cr alloys. Nevertheless, the Co-Cr castings, in general, posses less ductility than the Ni-Cr based alloys (see Table 1) [53].

Hero and colleagues [83] studied the ductility of some commercial cobalt-based dental casting alloys, and found substantial differences in the total elongation. Fracture analysis using the scanning electron microscope (SEM) revealed cracks nucleating from internal eutectic particles, and rapid propagation leading to an overall brittle fracture on alloys. It was also concluded that reducing the amount of carbon reduced the volume fraction of these eutectic particles, and this increased the ductility of the alloy. In part because of reductions in ductility with increasing carbon content, a solution-hardening mechanism is used to strengthen the PFM alloys, rather than the carbide formation used in partial denture restorations [53]. Heat treatments may also reduce the yield strength and ductility of cobalt-based alloys [53]. O'Connor and colleagues [62] found the castability of a Co-Cr alloy to be within the range of Ni-Cr alloys without Be additions. The thermal expansion coefficients of Co-Cr alloys, however, are often not as compatible with the porcelains as the Ni-Cr based alloys [54].

In general, in vitro electrochemical and dissolution studies have shown Co-Cr alloys to be more corrosion-resistant than the Ni-Cr family of alloys. Sarkar and Greener [85] showed significantly better corrosion resistance in

Ringer's solution for two cobalt-based casting alloys than a nickel-based casting alloy with less than 10% chromium. Holland [86] found a Co-Cr-Mo casting alloy to have substantially higher oxide breakdown potentials in NaCl and Fusayama's solution than a Ni High-Cr alloy with Mo additions. Wiegman-Ho and Ketelaar [87] showed that Co-Cr-Mo castings revealed substantially lower corrosion rates and higher polarization resistance values than Ni-Cr castings in an artificial saliva solution. Khamis and Seddik [88] found three Co-Cr-Mo alloys to not only have a higher corrosion resistance in an artificial saliva solution than the Ni-Cr alloy studied, but also to be electrochemically equivalent after multiple castings. Viennot and colleagues [89] studied the corrosion resistance of a Co-Cr-W to two palladium-silver (Pd-Ag) casting alloys in an artificial saliva solution. The study found that even though the Co-Cr alloy exhibited a lower polarization resistance compared with the Pd-Ag alloys, the Co-Cr alloy still exhibited excellent electrochemical properties. From these data, it was concluded that Co-Cr alloys are a suitable substitute for fixed prosthetics, and should no longer be limited to partial dentures and PFM restorations.

A dissolution study by Geis-Gerstorfer and colleagues [66] comparing the total substance loss of Ni-Cr-Mo to Co-Cr-Mo castings found that the Co-Cr-Mo alloys had a much smaller range of substance release compared with the Ni-Cr-Mo alloys over a 35-day period in a lactic acid-based NaCl solution. This study revealed that the dissolution curves for most of the Co-Cr-Mo castings flattened after the initial 1- to 2-week period, indicating a stable passive oxide layer. This initial increased metal ion release was attributed in part to a selective leaching of nonprecious metal components, thus creating a more corrosion-resistant alloy surface afterwards. Even though this increased initial release of metal ions could result in an allergic response, the reduced long-term release caused by the more stable passive oxide layer is less likely to produce long-term sensitivity issues. Another study by Okazaki and Gotoh [90] on the dissolution of a Co-Cr-Mo alloy in various electrolytes found the Co, Cr, and Mo release of the alloy to be very low in all solutions after a 1-week static immersion. Cr and Mo release increased from the alloy in electrolytes with pH less than 4. The absence of Ni in the composition of these Co-Cr castings, in combination with the low metal ion release rates, make them a viable alternative to patients that are sensitive to Ni. Because cobalt is also a known allergen, however, patients should be tested for cobalt allergies before substituting Co-Cr for Ni-Cr alloys, even if they are hypersensitive to nickel [54,91]. The very low ion release rates shown for Co metal ions in these studies suggest that a patient sensitivity reaction from Co-Cr castings would be unlikely.

Wrought cobalt-chromium materials

After WWII, soldiers came home complaining of their Elgin watches corroding, which led to the research creating Elgiloy (Elgiloy Specialty

Metals, Elgin, Illinois), a Co-Cr-Ni watch spring alloy that would later find its way into medical dental use [8,92]. Since that time, Co-Cr-Ni alloys have been used for over 50 years for orthodontic wires, and have superior fatigue resistance and a longer resilience compared with the stainless steel wires [8,93]. Co-Cr-Ni alloys can be cold-worked, and solution-hardened as well as precipitation-hardened [24]. As with stainless steel wires, heat treatments in a temperature range from 900°F to 1200°F have been shown to increase ductility of Co-Cr-Ni wires [93,94]. One manufacturer offers Elgiloy wires in four different tempers, which are defined as soft, ductile, semi-resilient, and resilient, and provide for a large range of ductility, formability, and resilience [9,95]. Ingram and colleagues [96] demonstrated less ductility in the Co-Cr-Ni wires before heat treatments compared with stainless steel orthodontic wires. After heat treatments, the Co-Cr-Ni wires increased greatly in ductility and have been shown to have similar mechanical properties and thus similar springback characteristics to the stainless steel wires (see Table 1) [24,96,97]. Asgarni and Brantley [98] found similar results and showed a 10% to 20% increase in elastic modulus and a 20% to 30% increase in yield strengths after heat treatments in Co-Cr-Ni wires. Although the heat treatments affect the ductility of Co-Cr-Ni wires, the stiffness of the alloy remains in the range of stainless steels [2,97]. Much like stainless steels, the soldering of some tempers of Co-Cr-Ni wires can be difficult [8,24,95]. Co-Cr-Ni wires in general are very resistant to corrosion and discoloration in the oral environment [8,24]. Sarkar and colleagues [27] found these Co-Cr-Ni wires to remain passive at potentials up to 300 mV versus SCE in an 0.1% NaCl solution, in comparison to Ni-Ti wires, which showed breakdown of passivity at these potentials. Overall, the superior corrosion and fatigue resistance of Co-Cr-Ni orthodontic wires compared with those of stainless steel make them a useful alternative.

In addition to wrought Co-Cr-Ni wires, Co-Ni-Cr-Mo wrought forgings are used for multicomponent load-bearing situations that exceed the mechanical properties of the Co-Cr castings. In dentistry, higher loaded implants, including blades, subperiosteals, bone plates, and screws, are often made of Co-Ni-Cr-Mo wrought forgings [11,53]. The increase in strength in these Co-Cr wrought alloys is often offset by a decrease in corrosion resistance compared with Co-Cr castings [99]; however, Speck and Fraker [100] found very similar oxide breakdown potentials for Co-Cr-Mo castings and Co-Ni-Cr-Mo forgings in Hanks solution at a neutral pH and physiological temperatures.

Titanium and titanium alloys

Titanium was discovered in the late 1700s and is the fourth most abundant metal in the earth's crust [101,102]; however, until the introduction of the Kroll process for extracting titanium in 1936, which was later patented in 1940 [103], titanium was not available to industry in abundant quantities or at a low enough cost [104]. Early animal implantation studies such as those by Bothe and colleagues [105] and Leventhal [106] found that the response of bone to titanium was better than that of the previous alloys of Vitallium and stainless steel, and that the weight loss of this new material in vivo was insignificant. These studies concluded that bone was actually "growing into contact" with titanium, thus making it ideal in the fixation of fractures. Starting in the early 1950s, Brånemark [107] took this concept further and found that titanium implanted to the upper and lower jaws of dogs could stand several years of loading without any change in stability, and without the tissue reactions shown to other materials at that time. His concept of intra-osseous implantation, where the bone was in a functional structural connection with a load-bearing implant, was later termed "osseointegration." Since that time, the use of titanium and its alloys is increasing in many dental applications, including implants, crowns, orthodontic wires, and partial denture frameworks.

Unalloyed titanium is commonly available in four different grades (grades 1–4) based on different allowable oxygen and iron content. Titanium goes through an allotropic transformation from the hexagonal close-packed α-phase, to a body-centered cubic β-phase at 885°C. This structure transition allows four different phase combinations of titanium alloys to be commercially available, including α, near-α, α/β, and β phases. In order for titanium to remain in the α/β and β phases, microstructural stabilizers are added to raise or lower the β-transformation temperature. Aluminum, carbon, nitrogen, oxygen, gallium, and tin are commonly added α-phase stabilizers to α/β alloys [8,53,108]. Molybdenum, cobalt, nickel, niobium, copper, palladium, tantalum, and vanadium are common β-phase stabilizers for α/β and β phase alloys [8,108]. With all of these alloy combinations possible, the most common titanium alloys used in dentistry are the α-phase commercially pure titanium, α/β Ti-6Al-4V, and β-phase Ti-Mo orthodontic wires. Titanium and its alloys are used in dentistry in both cast and wrought forms.

Cast titanium materials

Titanium castings have a higher production cost compared with that of the Ni-Cr and Co-Cr alloys, because of the need for specially developed casting systems to address certain physical and chemical properties [109]. Titanium reacts instantaneously with atmospheric gases such as hydrogen, oxygen, and nitrogen. Therefore, castings have to be performed in a well-controlled vacuum using argon or helium, because the reaction with oxygen leads to an alpha case layer on the surface that has an embrittling effect [53]. The molten titanium liquid may also react with the investment material itself unless the oxide of the investment is more stable than titanium oxide

[53,108,110]. Hero and colleagues [111] studied the effect of gas pressures in a two-chamber casting machine on titanium castings, and found lower pressures with nonvented molds to produce sounder castings than those at higher gas pressures. Even though titanium has an extremely low density that can cause problems with conventional gravity-based casting methodologies, centrifugal castings under a vacuum have produced better results [108]. For PFM restorations on pure titanium castings, the porcelain fusion temperature must be controlled to below 800°C to prevent phase transition from α to β-phase, and excessive oxidation that can weaken PFM bonding [108,112]. Porcelains must also be matched to the low thermal expansion coefficients of the titanium ($8-9.4 \times 10^{-6}/°C$) [8,108,112]. Atsu and Berksun [113] showed titanium PFM restorations to produce stronger metal-porcelain bonding in an argon atmosphere compared with a conventional vacuum in most cases. After 50 years of advancements in titanium casting techniques and equipment, consistent nearly precision castings are just recently attainable [53].

Titanium and its alloys provide strength, rigidity, and ductility similar to those of other dental alloys [53,108–110]. Whereas pure titanium castings have mechanical properties similar to Type III and IV gold alloys, some titanium alloy castings, such as Ti-6Al-4V and Ti-15V, have properties closer to Ni-Cr and Co-Cr castings, with the exception of the lower modulus (see Table 1) [53,108,114]. Even with these similar material strengths, the very low density of titanium makes the restoration lighter and more comfortable for the patient [108]. Titanium and its alloys provide excellent corrosion resistance to saline or acidic environments, and are considered among the most biocompatible implant metals. This excellent corrosion resistance, in combination with the lack of nickel and cobalt in the composition, make these alloys especially attractive for hypersensitive patients. Taira and colleagues [114] reported that cast pure titanium and Ti-6Al-4V, Ti-20Cu, Ti-15V, and Ti-30Pd alloys showed strong passivity, and were immune to corrosion attack in the oral environment. Gil and colleagues [115] found the Ti ion release from a commercially pure titanium casting to be very low in an artificial saliva solution at physiological temperatures. Even though titanium alloys are exceptionally corrosion-resistant because of the stability of the TiO_2 oxide layer, they are not inert to corrosive attack. When the stable oxide layer is broken down or removed and is unable to re-form on parts of the surface, titanium can be as corrosive as many other base metals [102]. Studies have shown that fluorides can infiltrate the titanium oxide layer, especially at low pH levels [102,116]. Siiril and Knnen [116], in a study on topical fluoride effects of commercially pure titanium, concluded that toothbrushes used in contact with titanium surfaces should be as nonabrasive as possible, and that long-lasting contamination with topical fluorides should be avoided. In addition, fretting or galling mechanisms can lead to breakdown of the oxide layer and corrosive attack in oxygen-deficient environments [11,102].

Wrought titanium materials

Since Brånemark discovered the osseointegration of titanium in the early 1950s and Linklow designed the screw and blade implants in the 1960s [107,117,118], commercially pure titanium and titanium alloys have been used for over a quarter century for endosseous and subperiosteal implants. The low elastic modulus of titanium is closer to that of bone than stainless steel or cobalt-chromium (see Table 1), which allows a closer matching between the implant and bone moduli at the interface. In 1977, the aerospace industry stabilized the β-phase of titanium at room temperature through the addition of molybdenum [2]. Shortly after that discovery, around 1980 Burnstone and Goldberg [24] introduced β-titanium orthodontic Ti-Mo wires.

Although processing of this Ti-Mo material involves the same high-reactivity problems described earlier for titanium and its alloys, these orthodontic wires finally provided a material with a modulus of elasticity in between that of nitinol and stainless steel or Co-Cr-Ni wires (see Table 1) [24]. This low modulus, combined with the resistance to fracture upon rather sharp bending, gives these Ti-Mo wires the highest formability of any of the orthodontic wires [8]. Ti-Mo wires in general have low stiffness, but are now available in a wider range of stiffness values [8,24,97,119]. The springback of Ti-Mo wires is higher than those for stainless steel wires [9]. These wires can also be highly cold-worked, have a true weldability, and are the only true nickel-free alternative among orthodontic wires [8,97]. The corrosion resistance of Ti-Mo orthodontic wires is also very good. Kim and Johnson [26] and Sarkar and colleagues [27] did not reach the oxide breakdown potentials of Ti-Mo wire during anodic polarization experiments in NaCl environments at potentials up to 2000 mV.

The mechanical and notched sensitivity [41], stress corrosion cracking [120,121], torsional [42], and smooth and notched corrosion fatigue properties [121,122] of a series of wrought titanium materials used for implants have been well-characterized in the laboratories of the author's institution. Of particular interest from these studies are the notched corrosion fatigue properties of Ti-6Al-4V ELI, which indicated it is much more notch-sensitive in fatigue than the single-cycle notch sensitivity tests had suggested. In contrast, the β-phase Ti-15Mo alloy was found to be the least sensitive to the presence of a notch or defect in fatigue, as expected because of its high ductility. Because of the stability of the same TiO_2 oxide layer, wrought titanium alloys in general exhibit superior corrosion resistance compared with cobalt chromium and stainless steel implant alloys. Fig. 3 shows unpublished cyclic polarization curves from the laboratories of the author's institution of three wrought titanium alloys, including α-phase commercially pure (CP) Ti-Grade 4, α/β Ti-6Al-4V ELI, and β-phase Ti-15Mo. All three alloys show low corrosion rates and similar oxide breakdown potentials, which far exceed those shown in the stainless steel, Ni-Cr, and Co-Cr

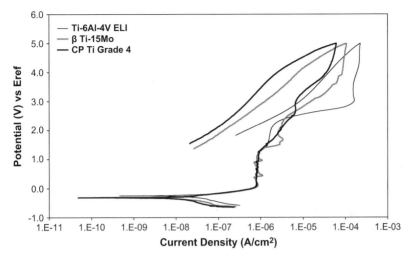

Fig. 3. Representative potentiodynamic curves of wrought titanium alloys in Ringer's solution at 37°C.

materials. There is also a lack of hysteresis between the forward and reverse voltage scans in any of the titanium alloys, indicating no evidence of pitting corrosion (see Fig. 3). Because the breakdown potential of titanium alloys in saline solutions is far superior to that seen in Co-Cr and stainless steel alloys, the likelihood of galvanic coupling between the titanium implant and other restorations of different nonprecious metals in the oral environment is a potential concern. Such a galvanic couple may accelerate the corrosion of the other metal, leading to increased metal ion release.

In addition to the various available casting techniques, single-unit dental crowns and multiple-unit bridges can also be machined from titanium billet on the Procera system (Nobel Biocare/University of Michigan, Ann Arbor, Michigan) invented by Andersson in the late 1980s [123]. This system uses computer-aided milling and electrical discharge machining, followed by the laser welding of multiple titanium restorations [108–110]. Although Boening and colleagues [124] found these milled crowns to show a high accuracy of fit in in vitro and in vivo studies, Leong and colleagues [125] reported no differences in marginal fit between cast and milled titanium crowns. In general, the low modulus of titanium requires lower machining speeds and cutting rates, sharp cutting tools, and additional cutting fluids [108]. Titanium also has a lower work hardening rate than 316L stainless steel, but can still be machined and polished to fine finishes. Watanabe and colleagues [126] studied the machinability of titanium and titanium alloys, and found the α/β-phase alloys to work best, followed by α phase alloys, and finally, β phase alloys.

Because of the unique biocompatibility of titanium, some do not consider these alloys to fall under the base metal classification [8]. Nevertheless, because of the lack of noble or precious metal components in the composition of the titanium alloys, they are classified here as a base metal alloy system. Regardless of the system of classification titanium falls under, this alloy system possesses unique corrosion and biocompatibility properties, which make it extremely useful as a biomedical implant material.

Nickel-titanium and shape memory alloys

In 1962, a space program metallurgist named Buehler developed an Ni-Ti alloy at the Naval Ordinance Laboratory. The alloy was given the name nitinol as an acronym for nickel titanium Naval Ordnance Laboratory [2,127]. Andreason first brought this material to dentistry for use as a new orthodontic wire around 1970 [2]. The name nitinol now includes a family of alloys, with slight variations in the percentages of nickel and titanium in the bulk compositions.

This alloy system exhibits shape memory effect (SME) and super-elasticity, giving it a unusual set of mechanical properties [127]. The SME is induced by changing the temperature of the alloy system. At the austenitic finish temperature, nitinol shows a stable body centered cubic (bcc) austenitic structure [127]. When the material is cooled through the temperature transition range (TTR), there is a change in the crystal structure to a twinned martensitic hexagonal structure, which can experience plastic deformation [53,127]. Additions of cobalt, and to some degree nickel, are often added to lower the TTR [53]. The microstructure transition can also be induced by applied stress. When stress is applied to the austenitic phase to the point of plastic deformation, a martensitic phase transformation occurs [127]. Instead of conventional plastic deformation, during this phase transformation stress does not increase with increased strain up to 8%, and is referred to as super-elasticity of the material [127].

Nitinol is more ductile in the martensitic phase, and plastic deformations that occur in this phase are fully recoverable by heating the alloy to the austenitic finish temperature [127]. In comparison to the stainless steel, Co-Cr-Ni, and Ti-Mo orthodontic wires, nitinol has a lower elastic modulus and yield strength that give it the highest springback value [24,53]. This high springback value allows the nitinol wire to use low forces to perform large deflections [9,24]. In addition, this alloy presents the highest resiliency of the four types of wire, meaning it can apply more moving force for tooth alignment [53]. Compared with the other orthodontic alloys, nitinol shows low formability, requires special techniques for bending, and is not recommended for bends with a small radius, because it readily fractures when bent sharply [9,24,53]. Because of its low formability, it is suggested that nitinol be used in preadjusted systems [9]. Also, because of the temperature-induced microstructure change, soldering or welding is not possible [53].

Mixed corrosion results have been found for nitinol exposed to saline environments. As noted earlier, Sarkar and colleagues [27] found nitinol to be less corrosion-resistant than the 18-8 stainless steel, Co-Cr-Ni, and Ti-Mo orthodontic wires in a 1% NaCl solution; however, studies such as Speck and Fraker [100] have shown Ni-Ti and Ti-Ni alloys to have a higher oxide breakdown potential (1100–1300 mV versus SCE) than 316L stainless steel, Co-Cr-Mo casting alloys, and Co-Ni-Cr-Mo wrought alloys in Hanks solution. Kim and colleagues also found nickel titanium wires to have higher oxide breakdown potentials (300–750 mV versus SCE) in NaCl solutions, and to exhibit lower levels of surface pitting than stainless steel wires. Unpublished cyclic polarization curves from the author's laboratory in Ringer's solution agree that nitinol has a higher breakdown potential than 316L, as shown in Fig. 4. Once the breakdown potential has been reached, however, the passive oxide layer breaks down because of pitting corrosion. The substantial pitting corrosion is shown in the polarization curve (see Fig. 4) as a large hysteresis between the forward and reverse voltage scans of the cyclic polarization curve, indicating a change in the materials response to the applied voltage in the reverse scan. This change in the voltage response of the material is caused by a change in surface area, and quite possibly localized surface and oxide compositions caused by selective leaching of specific elemental components of the material. When hypersensitive elements such as nickel are involved in such selective leaching processes, increased metal ion release into the surrounding tissues could possibly result in inflammatory tissue responses.

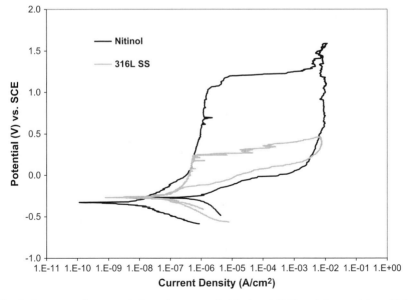

Fig. 4. Representative potentiodynamic curves of nitinol and 316L stainless steel in artificial saliva at 37°C.

In addition to orthodontic wires, Ni-Ti alloys have been used in dentistry for crowns and partial dentures, blade implants, and bone plates [127]. In general, the super-elastic Ni-Ti material provides properties in between those of the stainless steel, Co-Cr, and Ti-Mo materials used in orthodontics to complete the range of material properties available; however, the corrosion and even selective leaching of Ni ions caused by the high corrosion resistance of Ti make metal ion release from this alloy a potential concern for hypersensitive patients.

Summary

There have been many developments in the areas of nonprecious or base-metals used for dental restorations and implants in the last century. The wide array of materials available allows the clinician to choose the material and thus properties for the desired application. Titanium and Co-Cr materials in general provide superior corrosion resistance, especially for long-term exposure to the oral environment, whereas stainless steel and Ni-Ti materials provide substantial ductility and adequate corrosion resistance needed for other applications. With new materials continuing to emerge from most of these alloy systems, the future looks to present an even wider range of available material properties available to the clinician.

References

[1] Ring ME. A thousand years of dental implants: a definitive history   part 1. Compend Contin Educ Dent 1995;16(10):1060, 1062, 1064.
[2] Kusy RP. Orthodontic biomaterials: from the past to the present. Angle Orthod 2002;72(6): 501–12.
[3] Leinfelder KF. An evaluation of casting alloys used for restorative procedures. J Am Dent Assoc 1997;128(1):37–45.
[4] Morris HF, Manz M, Stoffer W, et al. Casting alloys: the materials and "the clinical effects". Adv Dent Res 1992;6:28–31.
[5] Paffenbarger GC, Caul HJ, Dickson MA. Base metal alloys for oral restorations. J Am Dent Assoc 1943;30:852–62.
[6] Sherman WO. Vanadium steel bone plates and screws. Surg Gynecol Obstet 1912;14(6):629–34.
[7] Strauss B. Steel alloy, 1,587,614. United States Patent Office; June 8, 1926.
[8] Anusavice KJ, Phillips RW. Phillips' science of dental materials. 11th edition. St. Louis (MO): Saunders; 2003.
[9] Kapila S, Sachdeva R. Mechanical properties and clinical applications of orthodontic wires. Am J Orthod Dentofacial Orthop 1989;96(2):100–9.
[10] Oh KT, Kim YS, Park YS, et al. Properties of super stainless steels for orthodontic applications. J Biomed Mater Res B Appl Biomater 2004;69(2):183–94.
[11] Lucas LC, Lemons JE. Biodegradation of restorative metallic systems. Adv Dent Res 1992; 6:32–7.
[12] TruChrome MSDS data sSheet. Rocky Mountain Orthodontics. Rocky Mountain Orthodontics. Available at: http://www.rmortho.com/products/info/MSDS/TruChrome%20 Stainless%20Steel.dot. Accessed September 5, 2006.

[13] Ratner BD. Biomaterials science: an introduction to materials in medicine. San Diego (CA): Academic Press; 1996.

[14] Shetty RH, Ottersberg WH. Metals in orthopedic surgery. In: Wise DL, editor. Encyclopedic handbook of biomaterials and bioengineering, vol. 1. New York: Marcel Dekker; 1995. p. 509–40.

[15] Moffa JP. Physical and mechanical pProperties of gold and base metal alloys. Presented at the Alternative to Gold Alloys in Dentistry. Bethesda (MD), January 24–26, 1977.

[16] Park JB, Lakes RS. Biomaterials: an introduction. 2nd edition. New York: Plenum Press; 1992.

[17] Morris HF, Asgar K, Rowe AP, et al. The influence of heat treatments on several types of base-metal removable partial denture alloys. J Prosthet Dent 1979;41(4):388–95.

[18] Elgiloy MSDS data sheet. Rocky Mountain Orthodontics: Rocky Mountain Orthodontics. Available at: http://www.rmortho.com/products/info/MSDS/Elgiloy.dot. Accessed September 5, 2006.

[19] Disegi J. AO/ASIF Materials Technical Commission. Titanium-6% aluminum-7% niobium implant material; AO/ASIF Materials Technical Commission, Switzerland; 1993.

[20] Disegi J. AO/ASIF Materials Expert Group. Wrought titanium 15% molybdenum implant material; AO/ASIF Materials Technical Commission, Switzerland; 2003.

[21] Goldberg J, Burstone CJ. An evaluation of beta titanium alloys for use in orthodontic appliances. J Dent Res 1979;58(2):593–9.

[22] Takahashi J, Okazaki M, Kimura H, et al. Casting properties of Ni-Ti shape memory alloy. J Biomed Mater Res 1984;18(4):427–34.

[23] Black J. Orthopaedic biomaterials in research and practice. New York: Churchill Livingstone; 1988.

[24] Burstone CJ, Goldberg AJ. Beta titanium: a new orthodontic alloy. Am J Orthod 1980; 77(2):121–32.

[25] Kusy R, Dilley G, Whitley J. Mechanical properties of stainless steel orthodontic archwires. Clin Mater 1988;3:41–59.

[26] Kim H, Johnson JW. Corrosion of stainless steel, nickel-titanium, coated nickel-titanium, and titanium orthodontic wires. Angle Orthod 1999;69(1):39–44.

[27] Sarkar NK, Redmond W, Schwaninger B, et al. The chloride corrosion behaviour of four orthodontic wires. J Oral Rehabil 1983;10(2):121–8.

[28] Lin MC, Lin SC, Lee TH, et al. Surface analysis and corrosion resistance of different stainless steel orthodontic brackets in artificial saliva. Angle Orthod 2006;76(2):322–9.

[29] Shin JS, Oh KT, Hwang CJ. In vitro surface corrosion of stainless steel and NiTi orthodontic appliances. Aust Orthod J 2003;19(1):13–8.

[30] Kerosuo H, Moe G, Kleven E. In vitro release of nickel and chromium from different types of simulated orthodontic appliances. Angle Orthod 1995;65(2):111–6.

[31] Staffolani N, Damiani F, Lilli C, et al. Ion release from orthodontic appliances. J Dent 1999;27(6):449–54.

[32] Seale NS. The use of stainless steel crowns. Pediatr Dent 2002;24(5):501–5.

[33] Threlfall AG, Pilkington L, Milsom KM, et al. General dental practitioners' views on the use of stainless steel crowns to restore primary molars. Br Dent J 2005;199(7):453–5 [discussion: 441].

[34] Peterson L. Fixation of bones by plates and screws. J Bone Joint Surg 1947;29:335–47.

[35] Howe GL, Greener EH, Crimmins DS. Mechanical properties and stress relief of stainless steel orthodontic wire. Angle Orthod 1968;38(3):244–9.

[36] Maijer R, Smith DC. Corrosion of orthodontic bracket bases. Am J Orthod 1982;81(1): 43–8.

[37] ASTM Standard Specification for wrought 18-chromium 14-nickel 2.5-molybdenum stainless steel bar and wire for surgical implants (UNS S31673) F138–00. Annual

book of ASTM standards. Section 13 - Medical devices and services, volume 13.01. West Conshohocken (PA): American Society for Testing and Materials; 2000.

[38] Zardiackas LD, Roach MD, Williamson RS, et al. Comparison of the corrosion fatigue of BioDur 108 to 316LS.S. and 22Cr-13Ni-5Mn stainless steels. In: Winters GL, Nutt MJ, editors. Stainless steels for medical and surgical applications. ASTM 1438. West Conshohocken (PA): ASTM International; 2003. p. 194–210.

[39] Fraker AC. Corrosion of metallic implants and prosthetic devices. Metals handbook. 9th edition, vol. 13. Metals Park (OH): ASM International; 1987. p. 1324–35.

[40] Beddoes J, Bucci K. The influence of surface condition on the localized corrosion of 316L stainless steel orthopaedic implants. J Mater Sci Mater Med 1999;10:389–94.

[41] Zardiackas LD, Roach MD, Williamson RS, et al. Comparison of the notch sensitivity and stress corrosion cracking of a low-nickel stainless steel to 316LS and 22Cr-13Ni-5Mn stainless steels. In: Winters GL, Nutt MJ, editors. Stainless steels for medical and surgical applications. ASTM 1438. West Conshohocken (PA): ASTM International; 2003. p. 154–67.

[42] Roach MD, McGuire J, Williamson RS, et al. Characterization of the torsional properties of stainless steel and titanium alloys used as implants. Proceedings of the 7th World Biomaterials Congress. Sydney (Australia); May 17–21, 2004.

[43] Zardiackas LD, Roach MD, Williamson RS, et al. Comparison of anodic polarization and galvanic corrosion of a low-nickel stainless steel to 316LS and 22Cr-13Ni-5Mn stainless steels. In: Winters GL, Nutt MJ, editors. Stainless steels for medical and surgical applications. ASTM 1438. West Conshohocken (PA): ASTM International; 2003.

[44] Roach MD, Williamson RS, Zardiackas LD. Comparison of the corrosion fatigue characteristics of 23Mn-21Cr-1Mo low nickel, 22Cr-13Ni-5Mn, and 18Cr-14Ni-2.5Mo stainless steels. Journal of ASTM International 2006;3(5):1–11.

[45] Hierholzer S, Hierholzer G. Internal fixation and metal allergie. Stuttgart (Germany): Thieme Medical Publishers; 1992.

[46] Hildebrand HF, Veron C, Martin P. Nickel, chromium, cobalt dental alloys and allergic reactions: an overview. Biomaterials 1989;10(8):545–8.

[47] Carpenter technology corporation BioDur 108 alloy data sheet. Available at: http://www.cartech.com/common/frames.html?http://cartech.ides.com/ListSearch.aspx?ST=DESC&i=101&leftn=sao_products&lefto=nav_tlo&lefti=nav_tlo3. Accessed September 5, 2006.

[48] Disegi JA, Eschbach L. Stainless steel in bone surgery. Injury 2000;31(Suppl 4):2–6.

[49] Gebeau RC, Brown RS. Tech spotlight—biomedical implant alloy. Advanced Materials and Processes 2001;159(9):46–8.

[50] Carpenter specialty alloys Corporation. BioDur 108 alloy data sheet. Reading (PA): CRS Holdings, Inc.; 2000.

[51] Ticonium. Available at: http://www.cmpindustry.com/company.asp. Accessed September 4, 2006.

[52] Touceda EG. Denture, 2,089,587. United States Patent Office; August 10, 1937.

[53] Craig RG, Powers JM. Restorative dental materials. 11th edition. St. Louis (MO): Mosby; 2002.

[54] Wataha JC, Messer RL. Casting alloys. Dent Clin North Am 2004;48(2):vii–viii, 499–512.

[55] Tucillo J, Cascone P. Composition and properties of noble and precious metal alloys. In: Smith DC, Williams DF, editors. CRC series in biocompatibility: biocompatibility of dental materials. Boca Raton (FL): CRC Press; 1982. p. 19–36.

[56] Baran G. Auger chemical analysis of oxides on Ni-Cr alloys. J Dent Res 1984;63(1):76–80.

[57] Baran GR. The metallurgy of Ni-Cr alloys for fixed prosthodontics. J Prosthet Dent 1983; 50(5):639–50.

[58] Bumgardner JD, Lucas LC. Surface analysis of nickel-chromium dental alloys. Dent Mater 1993;9(4):252–9.

[59] Covington JS, McBride MA, Slagle WF, et al. Beryllium localization in base metal dental casting alloys. J Biomed Mater Res 1985;19(7):747–50.

[60] Covington JS, McBride MA, Slagle WF, et al. Quantization of nickel and beryllium leakage from base metal casting alloys. J Prosthet Dent 1985;54(1):127–36.

[61] Roach MD, Wolan JT, Parsell DE, et al. Use of x-ray photoelectron spectroscopy and cyclic polarization to evaluate the corrosion behavior of six nickel-chromium alloys before and after porcelain-fused-to-metal firing. J Prosthet Dent 2000;84(6):623–34.

[62] O'Connor RP, Mackert JR Jr, Myers ML, et al. Castability, opaque masking, and porcelain bonding of 17 porcelain-fused-to-metal alloys. J Prosthet Dent 1996;75(4):367–74.

[63] Lee J, Lucas L, O'Neal J, et al. In vitro corrosion analyses of nickel-base alloys. J Dent Res 1985;63(DMG 1285):1–21.

[64] Meyer J. Corrosion resistance of nickel-chromium dental casting alloys. Corrosion Science 1977;17:971–82.

[65] Geis-Gerstorfer J, Passler K. Studies on the influence of Be content on the corrosion behavior and mechanical properties of Ni-25Cr-10Mo alloys. Dent Mater 1993;9(3):177–81.

[66] Geis-Gerstorfer J, Sauer KH, Passler K. Ion release from Ni-Cr-Mo and Co-Cr-Mo casting alloys. Int J Prosthodont 1991;4(2):152–8.

[67] Bumgardner JD, Lucas LC. Cellular response to metallic ions released from nickel-chromium dental alloys. J Dent Res 1995;74(8):1521–7.

[68] Wataha JC, Lockwood PE, Khajotia SS, et al. Effect of pH on element release from dental casting alloys. J Prosthet Dent 1998;80(6):691–8.

[69] Tai Y, De Long R, Goodkind RJ, et al. Leaching of nickel, chromium, and beryllium ions from base metal alloy in an artificial oral environment. J Prosthet Dent 1992;68(4):692–7.

[70] Winkler S, Morris HF, Monteiro JM. Changes in mechanical properties and microstructure following heat treatment of a nickel-chromium base alloy. J Prosthet Dent 1984;52(6):821–7.

[71] Marinello CP, Luthy H, Scharer P. Influence of heat treatment on the surface texture of an etched cast nickel-chromium base alloy: an evaluation by profilometric records. J Prosthet Dent 1986;56(4):431–5.

[72] Morris HF. Veterans Administration Cooperative Studies Project No. 147/242. Part VII: the mechanical properties of metal ceramic alloys as cast and after simulated porcelain firing. J Prosthet Dent 1989;61(2):160–9.

[73] de De Micheli SM, Riesgo O. Electrochemical study of corrosion in Ni-Cr dental alloys. Biomaterials 1982;3(4):209–12.

[74] Blanco-Dalmau L, Carrasquillo-Alberty H, Silva-Parra J. A study of nickel allergy. J Prosthet Dent 1984;52(1):116–9.

[75] Moffa JP. Biocompatibility of nickel based dental alloys. CDA J 1984;12(10):45–51.

[76] Jones TK, Hansen CA, Singer MT, et al. Dental implications of nickel hypersensitivity. J Prosthet Dent 1986;56(4):507–9.

[77] Haynes E. Metal alloy, 873,745. United States Patent Office; December 17, 1907.

[78] Lane JR. A survey of dental alloys. J Am Dent Assoc 1949;39:414–37.

[79] Prange CH. Cast metallic denture, 1,958,446: United States Patent Office; May 15, 1934.

[80] Gore D, Frazer RQ, Kovarik RE, et al. Vitallium. J Long Term Eff Med Implants 2005;15(6):673–86.

[81] Venable CS, Stuck WG. Electrolysis controlling factor in the use of metals in treating fractures. J Am Med Assoc 1938;111(13):1349–52.

[82] Venable CS, Stuck WG, Beach A. The effects on bone of the presence of metals based upon electrolysis. Annals of Surgery 1937;105(6):917–38.

[83] Hero H, Syverud M, Gjonnes J, et al. Ductility and structure of some cobalt-base dental casting alloys. Biomaterials 1984;5(4):201–8.

[84] Asgar K, Peyton FA. Effect of microstructure on physical properties of cobalt alloys. J Dent Res 1961;40(1):63–72.

[85] Sarkar NK, Greener EH. In vitro corrosion resistance of new dental alloys. Biomater Med Devices Artif Organs 1973;1(1):121–9.

[86] Holland RI. Corrosion testing by potentiodynamic polarization in various electrolytes. Dent Mater 1992;8(4):241–5.

[87] Wiegman-Ho L, Ketelaar JA. Corrosion rate studies: measurements of corrosion rates of some non-precious dental alloys in artificial saliva. J Dent 1987;15(4):166–70.

[88] Khamis E, Seddik M. Corrosion evaluation of recasting non-precious dental alloys. Int Dent J 1995;45(3):209–17.

[89] Viennot S, Dalard F, Lissac M, et al. Corrosion resistance of cobalt-chromium and palladium-silver alloys used in fixed prosthetic restorations. Eur J Oral Sci 2005;113(1): 90–5.

[90] Okazaki Y, Gotoh E. Comparison of metal release from various metallic biomaterials in vitro. Biomaterials 2005;26(1):11–21.

[91] Wiltshire WA, Ferreira MR, Ligthelm AJ. Allergies to dental materials. Quintessence Int 1996;27(8):513–20.

[92] Elgiloy. Available at: http://www.elgiloy.com/history.html. Accessed August 24, 2006.

[93] Fillmore GM, Tomlinson JL. Heat treatment of cobalt-chromium alloy wire. Angle Orthod 1976;46(2):187–95.

[94] Fillmore GM, Tomlinson JL. Heat treatment of cobalt-chromium alloys of various tempers. Angle Orthod 1979;49(2):126–30.

[95] Rocky Mountain Orthodontics. Product Catalog. Available at: http://www.rockymountai northodontics.com/assets/content.html. Accessed September 4, 2006.

[96] Ingram SB Jr, Gipe DP, Smith RJ. Comparative range of orthodontic wires. Am J Orthod Dentofacial Orthop 1986;90(4):296–307.

[97] Johnson E. Relative stiffness of beta titanium archwires. Angle Orthod 2003;73(3): 259–69.

[98] Asgharnia MK, Brantley WA. Comparison of bending and tension tests for orthodontic wires. Am J Orthod 1986;89(3):228–36.

[99] Devine TM, Wulff J. Cast vs. wrought cobalt-chromium surgical implant alloys. J Biomed Mater Res 1975;9:151–67.

[100] Speck KM, Fraker AC. Anodic polarization behavior of Ti-Ni and Ti-6A1-4V in simulated physiological solutions. J Dent Res 1980;59(10):1590–5.

[101] Disegi J. AO/ASIF Unalloyed tTitanium implant material; 1991.

[102] Tschernitschek H, Borchers L, Geurtsen W. Nonalloyed titanium as a bioinert metal—a review. Quintessence Int 2005;36(7–8):523–30.

[103] Kroll W. Method for manufacturing tTitanium and alloys tThereof, 2,205,854. Uniteds States Patent Office; June 25, 1940.

[104] Freese H, Volas M, Wood J. Metallurgy and technological properties of titanium and titanium alloys. In: Brunette DM, Tengvall P, Textor M, editors. Titanium in medicine: material science, surface science, engineering, biological responses, and medical applications. Berlin: Springer; 2001. p. 25–53.

[105] Bothe R, Beaton L, Davenport H. Reaction of bone to multiple metallic implants. J Surg Gynecol Obstet 1940;71(5):598–602.

[106] Leventhal GS. Titanium, a metal for surgery. J Bone Joint Surg 1951;33-A(2):473–4.

[107] Brånemark PI, Adell R, Breine U, et al. Intra-osseous anchorage of dental prostheses. I. Experimental studies. Scand J Plast Reconstr Surg 1969;3(2):81–100.

[108] Lautenschlager EP, Monaghan P. Titanium and titanium alloys as dental materials. Int Dent J 1993;43(3):245–53.

[109] Wang RR, Fenton A. Titanium for prosthodontic applications: a review of the literature. Quintessence Int 1996;27(6):401–8.

[110] Titanium applications in dentistry. J Am Dent Assoc 2003;134(3):347–9.

[111] Hero H, Syverud M, Waarli M. Mold filling and porosity in castings of titanium. Dent Mater 1993;9(1):15–8.

[112] Walter M, Reppel PD, Boning K, et al. Six-year follow-up of titanium and high-gold porcelain-fused-to-metal fixed partial dentures. J Oral Rehabil 1999;26(2):91–6.

[113] Atsu S, Berksun S. Bond strength of three porcelains to two forms of titanium using two firing atmospheres. J Prosthet Dent 2000;84(5):567–74.

[114] Taira M, Moser JB, Greener EH. Studies of Ti alloys for dental castings. Dent Mater 1989; 5(1):45–50.

[115] Gil FJ, Sanchez LA, Espias A, et al. In vitro corrosion behaviour and metallic ion release of different prosthodontic alloys. Int Dent J 1999;49(6):361–7.

[116] Siirila HS, Kononen M. The effect of oral topical fluorides on the surface of commercially pure titanium. Int J Oral Maxillofac Implants 1991;6(1):50–4.

[117] Linkow L. Intra-osseous implants utilized as fixed bridge abutments. Journal of Oral Implants and Transplants 1964;10:17–23.

[118] Ring ME. A thousand years of dental implants: a definitive history—part 2. Compend Contin Educ Dent 1995;16(11): 1132, 1134, 1136.

[119] McCracken M. Dental implant materials: commercially pure titanium and titanium alloys. J Prosthodont 1999;8(1):40–3.

[120] Williamson RS, Roach MD, Zardiackas LD. Comparison of stress corrosion cracking characteristics of CP Ti, Ti-6Al-7Nb, Ti-6Al-4V, and Ti-15Mo. In: Zardiackas LD, Kraay MJ, Freese HL, editors. Titanium, niobium, zirconium, and tantalum for medical and surgical applications (STP 1471). West Conshohocken (PA): ASTM International; 2006. p. 166–82.

[121] Zardiackas LD, Roach MD, Williamson RS. Comparison of stress corrosion cracking and corrosion fatigue (anodized and non-anodized grade 4 CP Ti). In: Zardiackas LD, Kraay MJ, Freese HL, editors. Titanium, niobium, zirconium, and tantalum for medical and surgical applications (STP 1471). West Conshohocken (PA): ASTM International; 2006. p. 202–14.

[122] Roach MD, Williamson RS, Zardiackas LD. Comparison of corrosion fatigue characteristics of CP Ti-grade 4, Ti-6Al-4V ELI, Ti-6Al-7Nb, and Ti-15Mo. In: Zardiackas LD, Kraay MJ, Freese HL, editors. Titanium, niobium, zirconium, and tantalum for medical and surgical applications (STP 1471). West Conshohocken (PA): ASTM International; 2006. p. 183–201.

[123] Andersson M, Bergman B, Bessing C, et al. Clinical results with titanium crowns fabricated with machine duplication and spark erosion. Acta Odontol Scand 1989;47(5):279–86.

[124] Boening KW, Walter MH, Reppel PD. Non-cast titanium restorations in fixed prosthodontics. J Oral Rehabil 1992;19(3):281–7.

[125] Leong D, Chai J, Lautenschlager E, et al. Marginal fit of machine-milled titanium and cast titanium single crowns. Int J Prosthodont 1994;7(5):440–7.

[126] Watanabe I, Kiyosue S, Ohkubo C, et al. Machinability of cast commercial titanium alloys. J Biomed Mater Res 2002;63(6):760–4.

[127] Thompson SA. An overview of nickel-titanium alloys used in dentistry. Int Endod J 2000; 33(4):297–310.

ELSEVIER
SAUNDERS

THE DENTAL
CLINICS
OF NORTH AMERICA

Dent Clin N Am 51 (2007) 629–642

Impression Materials: A Comparative Review of Impression Materials Most Commonly Used in Restorative Dentistry

Barry S. Rubel, DMD

Department of Care Planning and Restorative Sciences, University of Mississippi Medical Center School of Dentistry, 2500 North State Street, Jackson, MS 39216-4505, USA

Many impression materials are suitable for use in dentistry. Impression materials are used to record intraoral structures for the fabrication of definitive restorations. Accurate impressions are necessary for construction of any dental prosthesis. The relationship between static and mobile oral structures must be reproduced accurately for an optimum cast. Making a cast in gypsum materials from an impression of dental anatomy aids dentists in designing and constructing removable and fixed prostheses. The accuracy of these final restorations depends greatly on the impression materials and techniques. The more common types of impressions are used for fabricating diagnostic and master casts. Diagnostic casts are used to aid in treatment planning. Master casts are used for producing complete dentures, removable partial dentures, crowns, fixed partial dentures, and implant prostheses. Accurate impressions depend on identifying the applications that do or do not fit each material's characteristics. Materials used without adequate knowledge of their characteristics can impair a successful outcome. Often, the choice of impression materials depends on the subjective choice of the operator based on personal preferences and past experience with particular materials.

Ideal characteristics of impression materials

An ideal impression material should exhibit certain characteristics in the clinical and laboratory environment. Clinically, it should produce an

E-mail address: brubel@sod.umsmed.edu

accurate impression secondary to its adaptability to oral structures, have a consistency that is dimensionally stable to resist tearing but results in an atraumatic removal, set within a reasonable amount of time, demonstrate biocompatibility to include a hypoallergenic nature, and have a reasonable cost per use. In a laboratory setting, it should be dimensionally stable for accurate pouring of multiple casts and should not affect dimensional accuracy upon disinfection [1–4].

Common impression materials used in restorative dentistry

Impression materials that are currently popular include hydrocolloids, addition silicones, polyethers, and polysulfides. Some of the older impression materials (eg, zinc oxide eugenol impression paste, impression plaster, and impression compound) are still used in certain applications but are limited in use because they cannot be removed past undercuts without distorting or fracturing the impression [3]. All types of elastomeric impression materials undergo shrinkage caused by polymerization, and materials with reaction byproducts undergo additional contraction. The polysulfides and condensation silicones have the largest dimensional change during setting, in the range of −0.4% to −0.6%. The shrinkage is the result of the evaporation of volatile byproducts and the rearrangement of the bonds with polymerization. The addition silicones have the smallest change, approximately −0.15%, followed by the polyethers, approximately −0.2%. The contraction is lower for these two products because there is no loss of byproducts [2,3].

Depending on the manufacturer, many of the materials are available in cartridges for automixing and tubes or containers for hand spatulation. The automixing products require no mixing pads or spatulation, and training in their use is less time consuming. There may be less waste of material associated with automixing and providing a more bubble-free mix resulting in more accurate casts. Accessories such as intraoral tips, mixing tips, and various types of tray systems are also important when weighing the advantages and disadvantages of the delivery systems of impression materials.

Criteria used in evaluating impression materials

Properties and handling characteristics

The properties and handling characteristics of various contemporary impression materials are discussed in this section. The hydrophilic versus hydrophobic nature of materials is discussed as it relates to flow characteristics, which result in more bubble-free impressions. In recent years, dentists have turned toward using polyvinyl siloxanes and polyethers because of their improved physical and mechanical properties [1,5–7]. These properties include improved dimensional accuracy, stability, wettability, excellent elastic recovery, flexibility, ease of handling, tear strength, ability to produce multiple casts from one impression, and superior ability to reproduce detail.

Dimensional accuracy

With elastomeric impression materials such as polyvinyl siloxane, polyether, and polysulfide, the dimensional accuracy is usually time dependent, with greater dimensional accuracy occurring immediately after polymerization is complete but declining as the impression is stored for extended periods of time [5,7–9]. Polyvinyl siloxane and polyether impression materials remain dimensionally accurate for 1 to 2 weeks [5,7,8]. Polysulfide impression material is dimensionally accurate if poured within 1 to 2 hours of making the impression [5,7]. Practitioners should take this characteristic into consideration when selecting impression materials given the time available to the practitioner to pour casts during office hours.

Hydrophilic versus hydrophobic nature of impression materials. There are definite differences in the hydrophilic properties of elastomeric impression materials. Limitations of the polyvinyl siloxanes involve their hydrophobic nature [6,7,10–13]. Polyvinyl siloxanes are hydrophobic because of their chemical structure. They contain hydrophobic aliphatic hydrocarbon groups around the siloxane bond [2,3,13,14]. Polysulfides and polyethers are more hydrophilic. They contain functional groups that chemically attract and interact with water molecules via hydrogen bonding [13,15]. The hydrophilic nature of polyether impression material is manifested in carbonyl ($C=O$) and ether (C-O-C) groups, whereas polysulfide material has hydrophilic disulfide (-S-S-) and mercaptan (-S-H) groups [7,13,15]. The hydrophobic aspect of polyvinyl siloxane impression materials has an adverse effect on surface quality of the polymerized impression material [4,11,16–18].

Presence of moisture results in impressions with voids or pitted surfaces, and the detail reproduced is inferior. This result has been reported even with the new "hydrophilic" polyvinyl siloxane impression materials. These hydrophilic polyvinyl siloxanes have improved wettability [1,4,19,20], and they are only clinically acceptable under dry conditions [17]. The hydrophilization of polyvinyl siloxanes is enhanced with the incorporation of nonionic surfactants. They have a hydrophilic part and a silicone-compatible hydrophobic part. These surfactants act through a diffusion transfer of surfactant molecules from the polyvinyl siloxane into the aqueous phase. The surface tension of the liquid is changed, and increased wettability results [2]. When using polyvinyl siloxanes, moisture control is critical to ensure success for predictable clinical impression making. Because of their hydrophilic nature, using polyether and polysulfide impression materials is more compatible with the inherent moisture present in mucosal tissues [1–3,9].

If a comparison of the various categories of impression materials is made based on hydrophilic versus hydrophobic nature, wettability, the amount of detail reproduced, their dimensional stability, the rigidity of the material, the tear strength of the material, and the contact angle of the material, the selection of the right material is made easier. The hydrophilic nature of an impression material relates to its ability to work in a wet environment and still provide accuracy in impression making. If a material can tolerate some moisture, it is considered to be hydrophilic. Hydrocolloids would be considered the most hydrophilic. The hydrophobic nature of an impression material relates to its inability to work in a wet environment and still provide accuracy in an impression. Claims are made with respect to polyvinyl siloxane materials being hydrophilic, but in reality they are somewhat hydrophobic [1,4,8,20].

Dimensional stability

The dimensional stability of an impression material reflects its ability to maintain the accuracy of the impression over time [2]. These materials should have low shrinkage upon polymerizing and remain stable, which allows them to be poured days after making the impression. High impression dimensional stability materials usually can be poured within 1 to 2 weeks after the impression is made and still produce an accurate cast [2,3,5,8]. Materials with high dimensional stability are the polyethers and polyvinyl siloxanes, in contrast to alginate, which has a low dimensional stability. The polysulfides distort over time [14]. Because many dentists send their impressions to a laboratory to be poured, this characteristic should be considered when choosing an impression material [2,8].

Rigid impression materials require less support from trays. They distort less on pouring and make good bite registration materials [2,8]. They work well for implant impressions, in which posts must be transferred accurately [8]. They would be detrimental in making full arch impressions of periodontally compromised or mobile teeth. Polyethers and some polyvinyl siloxanes fall into this category.

Wettability (or flow characteristics)

Wettability of an impression material relates to the ability of the material to flow into small areas [2]. Impressions that wet the teeth well displace moisture and result in fewer voids. Materials with a high wetting angle do not flow easily into small crevices and are poor candidates for use in fixed prosthodontics. Materials with a low wetting angle flow extensively. Water is the ideal example of a material with a low wetting angle. Wettability results in fewer voids and less entrapment of oral fluids, providing more accurate impressions [2,4].

The ability of an impression material to reproduce minute detail in the area of 20 to 70 µm is necessary in the area of fixed partial dentures [3,17,18,21,22]. Impression materials with the ability to produce detail in the range of 100 to 150 μm work well and are acceptable in the areas of removable prosthodontics [23,24].

Elastic recovery

A set impression must be sufficiently elastic so that it will return to its original dimensions without significant distortion upon removal from the mouth [2]. Polyvinyl siloxane has the best elastic recovery, followed by polyether and polysulfide [2,8].

Flexibility

Flexible impressions are easier to remove from the mouth when set. Polyethers tend to be the most rigid impression materials [2]. Polyvinyl siloxanes are fairly stiff, and depending on the viscosity of the material, they flow readily to capture areas of detail [8]. Clinical studies have shown that the viscosity of the impression material is the most important factor in producing impressions and dies with minimal bubbles and maximum detail [2]. Accuracy of the impression is also affected when the percentage of deformation and the time involved in removing the impression are increased. In these instances, permanent deformation occurs relative to the type of elastomeric impression material used [2,8,14]. Alginate would be considered the most flexible of the impression materials, whereas polyethers would be considered the least flexible.

Ease of handling

Working times can be varied with respect to standard-set versus quick-set impression materials as prepared by various manufacturers [8]. Various viscosities and flow characteristics are also made available per individual manufacturer formulations.

Tear strength

The tear strength of an impression material relates to how resistant a particular material is to tearing after setting [2,3,25]. Where subgingival margins are concerned, this can be an important criterion. Polyethers are considered to have the highest tear strengths, whereas hydrocolloids have relatively low tear strengths [2,3]. Polysulfide impression materials have a high resistance to tearing but stretch and do not recover completely elastically [2,14].

Contact angle (and ability to reproduce detail)

Impression materials with low contact angle enable dental stone to flow easily, and relatively bubble-free casts are produced. Materials with high contact angle require more careful pour technique and attention to produce accurate casts [2]. Polyvinyl siloxane materials may require surfactants to lower the contact angle before pouring casts. Hydrocolloids, polyethers, and polysulfides have relatively low contact angles.

Miscellaneous

In addition to these criteria, the following criteria should be considered: how well a material is tolerated by patients, obtaining the best results for the least amount of expense, and occurrence of minimal changes when in contact with disinfection chemicals. Materials such as hydrocolloids, polyethers, and methacrylates may require specific disinfection protocols to prevent distortion of the material after setting [2,26–28].

Disinfection of impression materials. Impressions should be rinsed with water and then disinfected [29]. Diluted sodium hypochlorite (bleach 5.25%, 1:10 dilution, 10 minutes at 20°C) provides American Dental Association–accepted disinfection but not sterilization for all materials, except zinc-oxide eugenol paste. Glutaraldehydes are the disinfectant of choice for zinc oxide eugenol impression pastes [2,25].

Types and characteristics of specific impression materials

Irreversible hydrocolloids

When alginic acid (prepared from a marine plant) reacts with a calcium salt (calcium sulfate), it produces an insoluble elastic gel called calcium alginate. When mixed with water, the alginate material first forms a sol. The following chemical reaction forms a gel to create the set impression material. In an alginate impression compound, calcium sulfate dehydrate, soluble alginate, and sodium phosphate are in the powder. When water is added, calcium ions from the calcium sulfate dehydrate react preferentially with phosphate ions from the sodium phosphate and pyrophosphate to form insoluble calcium phosphate. Calcium phosphate is formed because it has a lower solubility; thus the sodium phosphate is called a retarder and provides working time for the mixed alginate. After the phosphate ions are depleted, the calcium ions react with the soluble alginate to form insoluble calcium alginate, which with water forms the irreversible calcium alginate gel. It is insoluble in water and its formation causes the material to gel [2,14].

After reviewing the types and characteristics of the most common impression materials, it becomes apparent that hydrocolloids have a high hydrophilic nature that allows this material to capture accurate impressions in the presence of some saliva or blood [14]. It has a low wetting angle so it easily captures full arch impressions. It has moderate ability to reproduce detail and costs relatively little compared with other impression materials. It is not accurate enough for fixed partial dentures but is used for partial framework impressions [2,23]. It has poor dimensional stability (imbibition or dessication is a problem), must be poured within 10 to 12 minutes of impression making or distortion becomes a major issue, and is good for only one pour per impression [8,25,30–33]. Impressions made in hydrocolloid are easier to remove than other materials and require rigid trays to prevent distortion in impression making and pouring of dental casts. Because the tear strength of hydrocolloids is low, it may capture subgingival contours and anatomy but may tear upon removal [2]. It is not as strong as polyethers or polyvinyl siloxane impression materials. It is relatively low cost and comes in flavors that are more patient friendly. Distortion can be a problem if disinfection guidelines are not strictly adhered to. Because hydrocolloids are hydrophilic, they swell if immersed in water or disinfectant [8,23,31]. It is recommended that a disinfectant spray be used while the impression is placed in a plastic bag for 10 minutes, at which time the impression is rinsed with water immediately and the cast poured [25,34]. If immersion disinfection (1% sodium hypochlorite or 2% potentiated glutaraldehyde) is performed (10–30 minutes), statistically significant dimensional changes are observed; these changes are on the order of 0.1%, and the quality of the surface is not impaired. (Such changes would be insignificant for clinical applications, such as study models and working casts.) Immersion disinfection also may differ between different brands of alginate with respect to different immersion systems, such as iodophor and glyoxal glutaraldehydes [2].

The setting reaction of hydrocolloids is not affected by latex proteins from gloves. Some water supplies contain large amounts of minerals that can adversely affect the accuracy and the setting time of alginate impression materials, however. If concerned about mineral content of local water supplies, distilled or demineralized water can be substituted [35]. Once set, hydrocolloid does not adhere to itself and cannot be used to border mold. A potential problem when using irreversible hydrocolloid is the tendency for this material to stick to teeth, which occurs when alginate radicals in the impression material form chemical bonds with hydroxylapatite crystals of the enamel. On removal of the impression, the alginate tears. Factors that may cause sticking of the alginate include polishing of teeth, which removes a thin film overlying the teeth and actually prevents the hydrophilic nature of this material from wetting the teeth and reproducing detail [23]. There is also a greater tendency for alginate to stick to teeth if they are dry. Dryness minimizes the moisture content of tooth surfaces and contributes to sticking of the alginate; ultimately, it leads to inaccurate cast pours. Finally, if repetitive impressions are made, the film over the teeth is lost and prevents satisfactory impression. Either placing a small amount of silicone lubricant over the teeth in a prophylactic paste or rehydrating through a rinse is necessary to produce a new film over the teeth for accurate impressions. Sometimes it is best to make another appointment for new accurate impressions within 24 hours or such a time so that this film layer will re-wet the tooth surfaces [35].

Polyethers

Polyethers consist of a base paste that is composed of a long-chain polyether copolymer with alternating oxygen atoms and methylene groups $(O-[CH_2]_n)$ and reactive terminal groups. Also present are fillers, plasticizers, and triglycerides. The catalyst paste has a cross-linking agent (aliphatic cationic starter) and filler and plasticizers. Polyethers involve the reaction of the polyether-containing imine ringed side chains with a reactant that opens the rings and causes chain lengthening and cross-linking to form a polyether rubber [2,14].

Polyether impression materials are moderately hydrophilic and capture accurate impressions in the presence of some saliva or blood. Because their wetting angle is low, they capture a full arch impression easier than with polyvinyl siloxanes [2]. Their ability to reproduce detail is excellent and they are dimensionally stable and allow multiple pours of accurate casts for 1 to 2 weeks after impressions are made, provided there is no tearing of the impression. They are rigid materials and may be more difficult to remove than polyvinyl siloxanes [2,14]. They do not tear easily (high tear strength), which enables the dentist to get good subgingival detail without tearing the impression on removal.

This material adheres to itself and can be used to border mold or make correctable impression techniques. Improved polyether formulations such as the "soft" polyethers are easier to remove, maintain proper rigidity for a wide range of applications, and capture fine detail even in moist conditions [36]. The snap-set behavior of the soft polyether materials allows the material to not start setting before the working time ends. When it does set, it does so immediately [23,36]. These characteristics make it highly desirable for clinical and laboratory use. Polyether has properties such that it can flow into critical areas with low pressure exerted, which results in accurate impressions and makes for fewer adjustments and remakes for the practice of dentistry. They are a superior material to hydrocolloids and somewhat better than polyvinyl siloxanes [2]. Because these materials are moderately hydrophilic, strict attention to disinfection guidelines is necessary to prevent swelling of the material. Spray with disinfectant for 10 minutes and rinse and dry immediately before pouring casts [34]. This material does taste bitter, although it is currently flavored to offset the taste. The setting times are relatively short (4–5 minutes), and the set is not altered or contaminated by latex gloves.

Polyvinyl siloxanes

Addition silicones (which are the most popular because no reaction byproducts are formed) involve the linking of a vinyl siloxane in the base material with a hydrogen siloxane via a platinum catalyst [1,2,8]. The reaction produces hydrogen, which is scavenged by the platinum. Viscosity is altered by changing the amount of silica filler, which produces either a putty or less viscous wash material. Vinyl polysiloxane silicones (also called addition silicones, polyvinyls, vinyls, and polyvinyl siloxane) are considered state-of-the-art for fixed partial denture impressions. They constitute the most widespread use of impression materials for fixed prosthetics [8]. They are virtually inert after set, and they can be trimmed and poured in any die material.

Before they set, however, they are susceptible to contamination. Because the addition silicones require a small amount of catalyst (platinum compound) to initiate the setting reaction, anything that interferes with the catalyst (preventing cross-linking of the material) causes the surface of the impression to remain tacky [2]. Polyvinyl siloxane contamination is usually a result of sulfur or sulfur compounds [2,8]. This is usually seen in the dental office in the form of latex gloves or rubber dams. Small amounts of sulfur interfere with setting of the critical surface next to the tooth and produce major distortion [3]. The preparation and adjacent soft tissues can be cleaned with 2% chlorhexidine to remove contaminants [2].

If wearing latex gloves, one should avoid touching the unset impression material, the teeth and adjacent gingiva, the interior of the tray, the mixing spatula or mixing pad, the end of a mixing tip, and the retraction cord. The way to avoid latex contamination is to wear polyethylene gloves over the latex gloves or not wear latex gloves during the impression procedures. Some vinyl gloves also may have the same effect because of the sulfur-containing stabilizer used in the manufacturing process [3]. Sulfur compounds can poison the platinum-containing catalyst in addition silicone impression materials and result in retarded or no polymerization in the contaminated area of the impression [2]. It has been reported that vapor given off by polysulfide impression material may cause contamination. It is a good idea not to store polyvinylsiloxane impression material close to polysulfide impression materials. Another source of contamination is the oxygen-inhibited layer on the surface of resin materials that appears immediately after curing. This thin layer causes impressions to remain tacky around new composite placed restorations [8].

Polyether and polysulfide impression materials also leave the mouth coated with a chemical film that inhibits polyvinyl siloxanes. If you make an impression with either of these two types of materials and then decide to make an impression with polyvinyl siloxane, it inhibits the set [1,8]. Polyvinyl siloxane materials are also thermally sensitive [8]. The warmer they are, the faster they set. If this material is overheated it may not recover to its normal setting time even after cooling, and it is recommended that this material be stored in a cool place and not in the sun (refrigerator or cool space). If cooled, the material sets slower. If kept in a refrigerator, it is advisable to let the material come to room temperature before use, otherwise it takes a longer time than normal to set. The material is thicker when it is cold and more difficult to express and mix [8].

Most impression materials require a 1:1 ratio of base to catalyst. More catalyst added also speeds the setting time. When using automix cartridges, it is recommended to extrude 0.25 inches of material and discard before placing the mixing tip to remove any contaminated material or material that has been exposed for long periods of time to the environment. Because some polyvinyl siloxane materials exhibit a phenomenon known as hydrogen out-gassing, if you pour casts too soon the stone captures these bubbles and produces a cast with pitted areas [3]. The newer materials are said to contain a proprietary component that eliminates hydrogen bubbles, but it is best to read the guidelines for pouring specific brands of polyvinyl siloxanes before pouring stone.

The newer materials are supposedly able to be poured in 5 minutes after the impression material is removed from the mouth. It is recommended that one wait at least 30 minutes for the setting reaction to be completed before the gypsum casts and dies are poured [3]. Epoxy dies should not be poured until the impression has stood overnight [2]. The difference in the delay with gypsum and epoxy is that gypsum products have a much shorter setting time than epoxy die materials. Some products contain a hydrogen absorber, such as palladium, and gypsum and epoxy die materials can be poured against them as soon as is practical [2].

Bubbles in the impression can occur when you spatulate and entrap air into the mix. Automixing cartridges tend to create fewer bubbles than hand spatulation. This is probably true with respect to any impression material when comparing hand spatulation to automixing. Polyvinyl siloxanes are generally hydrophobic. Aquasil (Caulk/Dentsply) is slightly hydrophilic [4,9,36]. Moisture from saliva or blood can interfere with accurate impressions. Loss of detail at impression margins is caused by moisture presence [3]. It has a moderately high wetting angle, which makes it a little more difficult to create an accurate full arch impression than with hydrocolloid, polyether, or polysulfide. It has an excellent ability to reproduce detail and is dimensionally stable, which allows multiple pours of accurate casts for several weeks after impressions are made if no tears are present in the material. The material is moderately rigid and can be more easily removed than polyether materials. Their tear strength is better than hydrocolloid but not as good as polyether [2,14]. They can be used with most disinfection protocols and may be cold sterilized without danger of distortion [34]. Note that addition silicones release hydrogen on setting and many require a 30-minute to 1-hour de-gassing period before pouring a master cast or the cast develops surface porosity.

There is a greater tendency to trap air bubbles when pouring stone because of its moderately high contact angle, so greater care is required when pouring stone [2]. This material comes in flavors and is not much of a problem from the standpoint of taste. The setting time is also relative short (4–5 minutes). However, contamination from the latex proteins in gloves may interfere with setting of this material. Most materials in this category do not adhere to themselves after they have set and would not be able to be used for border molding or correctable impression technique. Aquasil is an exception because it does adhere to itself after setting. Once set, polyvinyls are fairly inert, and there have been no reports of any disinfectants that damage them. High ambient room temperature does not distort them, and they can be trimmed and poured with any die material for casts.

Polysulfides

Polysulfide impression materials are supplied as two paste systems. The base consists of a polysulfide polymer (terminal/side chain −SH groups), titanium dioxide, zinc sulfate, copper carbonate, or silica. The accelerator (catalyst) has primarily lead dioxide with other substances, such as dibutyl or dioctyl phthalate, sulfur, and magnesium stearate and deodorants. The viscosity is altered by adding different amounts of titanium dioxide powder to the base. It sets by oxidation of the −SH groups, which results in chain lengthening and cross-linking and gives it elastomeric properties [2,14].

Polysulfide impression materials are generally low to moderately hydrophilic and make an accurate impression in the presence of some saliva or blood. Because the material has a low wetting angle it makes a full arch impression easier than with polyvinyl siloxanes or polyethers. It reproduces detail with excellent results but its dimensional stability is only fair [5,7–9, 14,37]. It may allow for more than one pour if it is not too thin in areas. It is not a rigid material, and impressions are easier to remove than with polyethers and polyvinyl siloxanes. It generally captures a subgingival margin upon impression without tearing on removal, which is much better than hydrocolloids or polyvinyls. It distorts from disinfection if not performed correctly because of its hydrophilic nature and may swell if placed in water or disinfectant for a period of time. Researchers recommend that it be sprayed with disinfectant for 10 minutes, rinsed, and dried immediately before pouring in dental stone [2,26]. It has a terribly bitter taste and is relatively inexpensive. It is not affected by latex gloves. Unfortunately, it does not adhere to itself, which makes it unavailable for border molding or correctable impression techniques.

Tissue conditioners (polyethyl or methyl methacrylates)

Tissue conditioners are composed of a powder that contains poly (ethyl methacrylate) and a liquid that contains an aromatic ester-ethyl alcohol (up to 30%) mixture. Tissue conditioners are soft elastomers. They show a weight loss of 4.9% to 9.3% after 24 hours as a result of the loss of alcohol. Within a few days, tissue conditioners become stiffer as a result of the loss of alcohol. Tissue conditioners are formulated to have specific viscoelastic properties. The viscoelastic properties are influenced by the molecular weight of the polymer powders and the power/liquid ratio [2]. Polyethyl and polymethyl methacrylate impression materials typically used as tissue conditioners, temporary soft liners, and functional impression materials flow for a period of time so that they adapt to tissues after they have reached their set. Because they have an extended flow period, they serve well as functional impression materials. They are all polyethyl or polymethyl methacrylate materials combined with an alcohol-based plasticizer [23].

The plasticizer makes each material unique and offers a different period of flow after the set. Plasticizers are moderately hydrophilic and make an accurate impression in the presence of some saliva or blood. Because of their low wetting angle, they easily capture full arch impressions. They are suitable for complete and partial dentures because they reproduce detail moderately. Their dimensional stability is fair and usually provides only one pour per impression. They have low rigidity and require rigid trays to support borders; otherwise they tend to distort. They are fairly easy to remove. These materials have low tear strength and usually tear on removal if not careful [2]. These materials are excellent for reline or rebase procedures in removable prosthetics [23]. As with all materials, there are learning curves with respect to working with these different tissue conditioners and other types of impression materials. They adhere to themselves and are excellent for border molding and correctable impression technique. They do not distort from water absorption, but because they are alcohol based, they distort easily when exposed to alcohol-based disinfectants, such as Lysol [2,3,25,34]. For the most part they have a neutral taste.

Summary

Dentists have relied on impression materials for various uses, including fabricating dental prostheses, serving as temporary liners, and serving as bite registration materials. The materials that have received a lot of attention because of their physical and handling properties include the irreversible hydrocolloids, polyethers, polyvinyls, and polysulfides.

The polyvinyls (addition silicones) and the polyethers account for a major portion of the market used as impression materials in fabricating fixed partial dentures, removable appliances, and implant prostheses. The hydrophilic addition silicones and polyethers flow easily, result in fewer retakes, and produce more bubble-free casts when used under appropriate guidelines. The polyvinyl siloxane materials are intrinsically hydrophobic (water repellent) by nature, so they must be made hydrophilic by adding surfactants. When these surfactants come into contact with moisture, it has to migrate to the surface, which prevents the hydrophilicity from fully developing during working and setting times and can result in voids and inaccurate impressions. A dry field is critical for their use. Polyether is hydrophilic by nature of its chemical makeup, and moisture does not interfere as much with achieving void-free impressions.

The condensation silicones, polysulfides, and irreversible hydrocolloids have qualities that make them more sensitive with respect to handling considerations and mix-and-pour techniques because they exhibit more changes over time after setting, which may affect accuracy in detail reproduction. The polyvinyls and polyethers are more stable to deformation after setting has occurred. All have specific protocols for disinfecting that must be followed to prevent distortion of the material before pouring casts; however, the polyvinyls seem to be most impervious to different disinfection protocols.

References

[1] Mandikos MN. Polyvinylsiloxane impression materials: an update on clinical use. Aust Dent J 1998;43:428–34.

[2] Craig RG, Robert G. Restorative dental materials. 11th edition. Elsevier 2002. p. 12.

[3] Anusavice KJ, Kenneth J. Phillips' science of dental materials. 11th edition. Elsevier 2003. p. 12.

[4] Panichuttra R, Jones RM, Goodacre C, et al. Hydrophobic poly(vinyl siloxane) impression materials: dimensional accuracy, wettability, and effect on gypsum hardness. Int J Prosthodont 1991;4(3):240–8.

[5] Shen C. Impression materials. In: Anusavice KJ, editor. Phillip's science of dental materials. 11th edition. Philadelphia: Saunders; 2003. p. 210–30.

[6] Craig RG, Urquiola NJ, Liu CC. Comparison of commercial elastomeric impression materials. Oper Dent 1990;15:94–104.

[7] Williams PT, Jackson DG, Bergman W. An evaluation of the time-dependent dimensional stability of eleven elastomeric impression materials. J Prosthet Dent 1984;52:120–5.

[8] Donovan JE, Chee WW. A review of contemporary impression materials and techniques. Dent Clin North Am 2004;48(2):445–70, vi–vii.

[9] Derrien G, Le Menn G. Evaluation of detail reproduction for three die materials by using scanning electron microscopy and two-dimensional profilometry. J Prosthet Dent 1995;74: 1–7.

[10] Pratten DH, Craig RG. Wettability of a hydrophilic addition silicone impression material. J Prosthet Dent 1989;61:197–202.

[11] Mc Murry J. Fundamentals of organic chemistry: their correlation with chemical structure. 4th edition. Pacific Grove (CA): Brooks/Cole Publishing; 1998. p. 36–45.

[12] Johnson GH, Lepe X, Aw TC. The effect of surface moisture on detail reproduction of elastomeric impressions. J Prosthet Dent 2003;90:354–64.

[13] Peutzfeldt A, Asmussen E. Impression materials: effect of hydrophilicity and viscosity on ability to displace water from dentin surfaces. Scand J Dent Res 1988;96:253–9.

[14] Giordano R. Impression materials: basic properties. Gen Dent 2000;48:510–6.

[15] Chong YH, Soh G, Setchell DJ, et al. Relationship between contact angles of die stone on elastomeric impression materials and voids in stone casts. Dent Mater 1990;6:162–6.

[16] Takahashi H, Finger WJ. Dentin surface reproduction with hydrophilic and hydrophobic impression materials. Dent Mater 1991;7:197–201.

[17] Shillingburg HT, Herbert T. Fundamentals of fixed prosthodontics. 3rd edition. Quintessence; 1997. p. 299–300.

[18] Petrie CS, Walker MP, O'Mahony AM, et al. Dimensional accuracy and surface detail reproduction of two hydrophilic vinyl polysiloxane impression materials tested under dry, moist and wet conditions. J Prosthet Dent 2003;90:365–72.

[19] Boening KW, Walter MH, Schuette U. Clinical significance of surface activation of silicone impression materials. J Dent 1998;26:447–52.

[20] Chee WW, Donavan TE. Polyvinylsiloxane impression materials: a review of properties and techniques. J Prosthet Dent 1992;68:728–32.

[21] Bindl A, Mormann WH. Marginal and internal fit of all-ceramic CAD/Cam crown copings on chamfer preparations. J Oral Rehabil 2005;32(6):441–7.

[22] Boeckler AF, Stadler A, Jurgen M. The significance of marginal gap and overextension measurement in the evaluation of the fit of complete crowns. J Contemp Dent Pract 2005;6(4): 1–12.

[23] Phoenix RD, Rodney D. Stewart's clinical removable partial prosthodontics. 3rd edition. Quintessence; 2002. p. 162–7.

[24] Craig RG. Restorative dental materials. 6th edition. The C.V. Mosby Company; 1980. p. 203.

[25] Little J. Dental management of the medically compromised patient. 6th edition. Elsevier; 2002. p. 545–7.

[26] Adabo GL, Zanarotti E, Fonseca RG, et al. Effect of disinfectant agents on dimensional stability of elastomeric impression materials. J Prosthet Dent 1999;81(5):621–4.

[27] Lepe X, Johnson GH. Accuracy of polyether and addition silicone after long-term immersion disinfection. J Prosthet Dent 1997;78(3):245–9.

[28] Pratten DH, Covey DA, Sheats RD. Effect of disinfectant solutions on the wettability of elastomeric impression materials. J Prosthet Dent 1990;63(2):223–7.

[29] Leung RL, Schonfeld SE. Gypsum casts as a potential source of microbial cross-contamination. J Prosthet Dent 1983;49:210.

[30] Combe EC, Burke FJT, Douglas WH. Dental biomaterials. Boston: Kluwer; 1999:294.

[31] Miller MW. Syneresis in alginate impression materials. Br Dent J 1975;139:425–30.

[32] Osborne J, Lammie GA. The manipulation of alginate impression material. Br Dent J 1954; 96:51–8.

[33] Rudd KD, Morrow RM, Rhodes JE. Dental laboratory procedures. Vol. 3: Removable partial dentures. St. Louis (MO): Mosby; 1986. p. 6.

[34] Cottone JA, Molinari JA. State-of-the-art infection control in dentistry. J Am Dent Assoc 1991;122(9):33–41.

[35] Skinner EW, Carlisle FB. The use of alginate impression materials in the Sears' hydrocolloid impression technique. J Prosthet Dent 1956;6:405–11.

[36] Klettke Th, Kuppermann B, Fuhrer C, et al. Hydrophilicity of precision impression materials during working time. Istanbul (Turkey): CED/IADR; 2004.

[37] Ciesco JN, Malone WF, Sandrik JL, et al. Comparison of elastomeric impression materials used in fixed prosthodontics. J Prosthet Dent 1981;45(1):89–94.

ELSEVIER
SAUNDERS

Dent Clin N Am 51 (2007) 643–658

THE DENTAL
CLINICS
OF NORTH AMERICA

Dental Cements for Definitive Luting: A Review and Practical Clinical Considerations

Edward E. Hill, DDS, MS

Department of Care Planning and Restorative Sciences, University of Mississippi Medical Center School of Dentistry, 2500 North State Street, Jackson, MS 39116, USA

A dental cement used to attach indirect restorations to prepared teeth is called a luting agent [1]. Luting agents may be definitive or provisional, depending on their physical properties and the planned longevity of the restoration. A 2001 survey indicated that many clinicians are now exclusively using newer resin-modified glass-ionomer and resin luting materials based primarily on ease of use, reasonable retention, and low to no postoperative sensitivity [2]. The literature continues to repeat that "No available product satisfies the requirements for an ideal luting agent and comprehensive patient care requires several materials.... the best choice is not always easy" [3]. The purpose of this article is to provide a clinically relevant discussion of definitive luting agents, in order to enhance the dentist's ability to make intelligent cementation choices and application.

Luting agent requirements

In the simplest view, a luting agent has to hold an indirect restoration in place for an indefinite period of time, and fill the gap at the tooth-restoration interface. Basic mechanical, biological, and handling requirements must be met by the cement [4]:

It must not harm the tooth or tissues.
It must allow sufficient working time to place the restoration.
It must be fluid enough to allow complete seating of the restoration.
It must quickly form a hard mass strong enough to resist functional forces.

E-mail address: eehill@sod.umsmed.edu

It must not dissolve or wash out, and must maintain a sealed, intact restoration.

All current definitive luting materials satisfy these requirements somewhat, and all have been used with clinical success [5]. Rosentiel and colleagues [3] described the ideal luting agent as being biocompatible, preventing caries or plaque, resistant to microleakage, having sufficient strength to resist functional forces over the lifetime of the restoration, having low water solubility and no water sorption, being adhesive, radiopaque, esthetic, easy to manipulate, low in cost, and having low viscosity at mixing.

Comparative data of physical testing for various luting materials can be confusing to many practitioners (ie, laboratory data do not always predict clinical performance) [6]. Although each has unique physical properties based on composition, it is very important to appreciate that those properties can vary considerably if the materials are not manipulated and used according to the manufacturer's directions (Table 1) [7].

Classifications

Almost all cements are formed by the interaction of a powder capable of releasing cations into acid solution (a base) and a liquid (an acid) capable of liberation of cement-forming cations, and having acid anions that form stable complexes with those cations to yield a salt. The set cement is thus a salt hydrogel matrix surrounding unreacted powder. Typically, the matrix is the weakest and most soluble component of the set cement. Those materials are classified as AB (acid-base) cements, as opposed to cements formed by the polymerization of macromolecules. All current cements fall into the AB category except for resins (and possibly compomers) [8].

The literature varies considerably on the classification and discussion of cements. Craig [9] followed a traditional method of classifying cements according to chief ingredients (ie, zinc phosphate, zinc silicophosphate, zinc oxide-eugenol, zinc polyacrylate, glass-ionomer, and resin), whereas O'Brien [10] classified dental cements by matrix bond type (ie, phosphate, phenolate, polycarboxylate, resin, and resin-modified glass-ionomer). Donovan simply divided cements into conventional (zinc phosphate, polycarboxylate, glassionomer) and contemporary (resin-modified glass-ionomers, resin) based on knowledge and experience using these materials [6].

Retention and bonding

Mechanical interlocking with rough surfaces on a parallel wall preparation is the principal means of retention for luting cement, regardless of chemical composition [5]. Schillingburg and colleagues [11] described cement luting mechanisms as nonadhesive, micromechanical, and molecular

Table 1
Properties of luting cements for comparison

	Setting time (minutes)	Strength (MPa) compressive	tensile	Solubility (weight % at 24 hours)	Modulus of elasticity (GPa)	Bond to tooth	Excess removal (set)	Fluoride release
Zinc phosphate	5–9	96–133	3.1–4.5	0.2 max	13	no	easy	no
Zinc polycarboxylate	7–9	57–99	3.6–6.3	0.06	5–6	some	some	no
Glass-ionomer	6–8	93–226	4.2–5.3	1	7–8	chemical	fair	yes
Resin-modified glass-ionomer	5.5–6	85–126	13–24	0.7–0.4	2.5–7.8	chemical	difficult	yes
Resin	4+	180–265	34–37	0.05	4–6	micro-mechanical	very difficult	no
Adhesive resin	–	52–224	37–41	–	1.2–10.7	micro-mechanical	very difficult	no

Data from Craig RG, Powers JM. Restorative dental materials. 11th edition. St Louis: Mosby; 2002. p. 594–634; and O'Brien W. Dental materials and their selection. 3rd edition. Chicago: Quintessence; 2002. p. 133–55.

adhesion. In nonadhesive bonding, cement fills the restoration/tooth gap and holds by engaging in small surface irregularities (all cements do this). In micromechanical bonding, surface irregularities are enhanced through air abrasion or acid etching to provide larger defects for the cement to fill, which works well for materials with high tensile strength (resins or resin-modified glass-ionomers). Molecular adhesion results from bipolar, Van der Waals forces, and weak chemical bond formation between cement and tooth structure (polycarboxylate and glass-ionomer).

In direct restoration, retention frequently parallels cement mechanical properties (compressive, shear, tensile strengths, and elastic modulus). But a clinician who chooses a luting agent based solely on mechanical properties may not always be totally correct, because tooth preparation and restoration design have a significant influence on restoration retention and the demands placed on the cement layer [5,12].

Definitive luting agents—conventional

Zinc phosphate

Zinc phosphate is the oldest luting cement (introduced in the 1800s), and has been used with a high degree of success for metal, metal-ceramic, and porcelain restorations; it is the standard to which other cements are compared. It is the classical AB cement, being supplied as a separate powder/liquid system—the powder approximately 90% zinc oxide (ZnO) and the liquid approximately 67% buffered phosphoric acid. Aluminum (1%–3%) in the liquid is needed for the cement-forming reaction, and water (~33%) partially controls the reaction rate. The liquid bottle should remain closed unless dispensing to prevent water loss by evaporation, and batches of powder and liquid are matched by the manufacturer, so items should not be interchanged. Many modifications have been tried with no significant improvement in properties [8]; silicate was added to provide a more translucent material for luting porcelain jacket crowns [9].

Zinc phosphate should be mixed on a cool, dry, glass slab to slow the exothermic reaction, allowing maximum powder to be brought into the mix while controlling the viscosity. Powder should be incorporated into the liquid over 60 to 90 seconds in several small increments, by spreading the mix over a broad area with a metal spatula. The correct mix consistency for optimal strength and to allow complete seating of the restoration is important—strength is linear to powder/liquid ratio, but viscosity also increases [10]. It should be fluid, yet string about 2 to 3 cm when lifting the spatula from the mix [9]. The restoration should be seated within 3 to 5 minutes with firm, steady pressure, which should be maintained several minutes until the initial set has occurred [11].

Zinc phosphate functions by nonadhesive bonding, quickly reaching maximal physical properties within 24 hours. Compressive strength is very high, tensile strength low compared with other available cements. The set material is brittle and stiff, having a high elastic modulus. Early solubility is high, but falls rapidly as the cement ages, yet can be significant, especially in an acid environment [8]. Minimal exposure to oral fluids is necessary (ie, well-fitting restoration margins are required) and caution is recommended for use in patients who have a very acidic diet, or who have acid reflux problems. At cost per unit dose, zinc phosphate is the least expensive luting agent.

The pH of zinc phosphate is very low (less than 4) at 1 hour after delivery, but reaches neutrality by 48 hours. Its use in not recommended for deep preparations, or if pulpal irritation is a concern (because of low pH and hydraulic seating pressure). Some have recommended use of a cavity varnish [8,9] or calcium hydroxide liquid over the preparation before cementation, if less than 1 mm of dentin remains between the pulp and cement [9,13]. Use of a resin-based sealer is not recommended because of a marked reduction in retention [14]. Because of early strength and acceptable physical properties, extremely low cost, and lack of technique sensitivity, zinc phosphate remains a good clinical choice for luting metal, well-fitting metal-ceramic restorations, long-span fixed partial dentures, and cast dowel (post) cores [6].

Polycarboxylate

Zinc polycarboxylate cement was introduced in 1968 by Smith [15] as the first luting cement that would adhere to tooth structure. As a hybrid of zinc phosphate, the AB cement powder is mostly zinc oxide (10% magnesium oxide) and the liquid a 30% to 43% solution of high molecular weight poly(alkenoic acids). When hand-mixed in correct proportions, the mix is somewhat thicker than zinc phosphate because of the viscous nature of the organic acids, but it is pseudo-plastic, and flows readily upon seating of the restoration because of shear thinning [5,8]. The cement should appear glossy when used; if dull, it may be too thick to allow proper seating of the restoration [9]. Working time (4–6 minutes) can be prolonged by cooling the mixing slab, and seating of the restoration should be with prolonged, firm pressure, as with zinc phosphate.

Polycarboxylate cement reaches early end strength, but values cited in the literature are quite variable, depending on testing conditions and parameters [8]. In general, the compressive strength for polycarboxylate is one half to two thirds that of zinc phosphate, and the tensile strength one third more. The modulus of elasticity (stiffness) is approximately one third of that for zinc phosphate, giving a material that can display significant plastic deformation upon loading [9]. For that reason, it is not recommended for long-span fixed partial dentures, or where subjected to high functional stress [16]. Many feel that cement modulus of elasticity should match that of dentin; therefore zinc phosphate and polycarboxylate deviate from ideal by being too stiff and too flexible respectively. Solubility is comparable to zinc phosphate, with acidic conditions greatly increasing the erosion of the cement [8].

Two desirable properties of this luting agent are a degree of adhesion to the preparation and favorable biocompatibility. Chemical adhesion to tooth occurs through interaction of free carboxylic groups to calcium [10,16], so bonding is best to enamel, and requires a clean, uncontaminated surface [5,10]. Adhesion to tooth should not be an excuse to overlook primary retention and resistance factors in the preparation and the importance of a well-fitting restoration, because interfacial adhesive failures can occur at the cement-metal interface [16]. Although more acidic than zinc phosphate when mixed, polycarboxylate pH rises rapidly, and penetration of the large organic acid molecules into dentin tubules is minimal [9]. Therefore the pulpal response is mild; biocompatibility is considered to be excellent [5]. Encapsulated polycarboxylate (Duralon, 3M ESPE, St. Paul, Minnesota) is now available, which simplifies mixing while improving consistency.

Glass-ionomer (glass polyalkenoate)

Glass-ionomer cement, introduced in 1969 by Wilson and Kent, was originally know as ASPA (aluminosilicate polyacrylic acid) based on the main constituents of the AB cement. It was developed from the desire to have a luting agent with the fluoride release/translucency of dental silicate cement and the adhesion to tooth of polycarboxylate cement. The International Standards Organization officially uses the name "glass polyalkenoate cement," with the term "glass-ionomer" considered as generic, and covering a larger group of cements with similar compositions [8].

The powder is usually a calcium aluminosilicate glass (some mixtures replace calcium with strontium or lanthanum), and contains fluoride to help control cement formation and modify properties. The liquid is dilute poly(alkenoic acids)(poly(acrylic acid), itaconic acid, maleic acid, plus other minor organic acids, although the acid components may be dried and combined with the powdered glass, to be later mixed with water or dilute tartaric acid solution [8]. Dispensing should be exactly to manufacturer instructions, because too much powder will reduce the working time while increasing viscosity; too little powder will significantly reduce physical properties. Most manufacturers offer encapsulated ingredients for machine mixing, which simplifies and expedites mixing. Mount [17] recommended periodically checking the quality of glass-ionomer mixing by using a loss-of-gloss technique to insure consistent, predictable results. Typically, mixing time is ten seconds at 3000 cycles/min; either too long or too short of a mixing cycle can affect working time and physical properties markedly [18].

Working time for glass-ionomer cement is shorter than that for zinc phosphate or polycarboxylate ($\sim$2–3 1/2 min.). The material should have a glossy surface when the restoration is placed, and should flow easily to allow complete seating without the firm, sustained pressure required for the previously discussed luting agents. A dull finish on the surface of the excess occurs rapidly with the material achieving a sudden "snap set" [17]. Because of the snap set, quickness must be exercised to insure complete seating for all restorations. Prior to cementation, the tooth surface should be clean and dry but not dehydrated, with the smear layer retained. To reduce potential postoperative sensitivity, the use of a resin-based sealer, which also enhances retention, has been recommended [14].

When to remove the excess and how to expose the glass-ionomer to the oral environment has been somewhat confusing. Water balance is important in the newly placed cement, because it contains water and releases water during the setting process. As with any AB cement, contamination by saliva must be avoided for several minutes to prevent loss of material by erosion caused by early solubility. Wilson and Nicholson [8] recommended temporary protection with a varnish after bulk removal, because some of the ions are still in soluble form while the matrix is forming. Curtis and colleagues [19] found that leaving excess glass-ionomer cement expressed during restoration seating undisturbed for 10 minutes prevents any significant erosion in a wet field; in contrast, keeping the exposed cement dry for too long risks possible dehydration and microcracking. Applying petroleum jelly to the exposed glass-ionomer cement margin after bulk removal has been suggested as a simple solution to maintain water balance [20]. Mount [17] discussed this dilemma, and commented that newer glass-ionomer luting cements are fast-setting and have relatively high resistance to water within 5 minutes, so that it is unnecessary to use a waterproof varnish or resin sealer to cover the exposed cement, as previously recommended. Dehydration remains a problem, so isolation from the oral environment for longer than 10 minutes is not recommended.

Although glass-ionomer luting cement has a snap set, the chemistry of the entire setting reaction is quite complex, and has been divided into at least four overlapping stages, which begin at mixing and take several months to reach completion [8,17]. Patients should limit heavy functional stress on restorations luted with glass-ionomer cements for several days to allow physical properties of the cement to fully develop. Laboratory tests have reported compressive strength and crown retention results higher than zinc phosphate; microleakage studies give variable comparisons, and antibacterial properties are considered slightly better [3]. Shelf life may be an issue, because viscosity has been shown to increase after 24 months [4]. The modulus of elasticity for glass-ionomer is less than that for zinc phosphate, and may be a concern for usage with multiple abutment or long-span, fixed partial dentures, or in areas of excessive masticatory stress [16].

Chemical adhesion to tooth structure by chelation with calcium and phosphate ions in dentin and enamel, good translucency, and slow, long-term fluoride-release–enhancing cariostatic potential are all factors that have made glass-ionomer an extremely popular definitive luting agent [16,17]. Fluoride release has been shown to be pH-dependent (being greater at lower pH values), plus glass-ionomer cement displays fluoride uptake (fluoride recharge) when exposed to topical fluoride. Selection of this material as a luting agent may be an important issue for the patient who has high caries potential [21].

Early concerns and reports of post-cementation sensitivity when using glass-ionomer cements have largely been dismissed as being multifactorial in origin [16], although studies concerning pulpal reactions to these materials are highly variable in results [13]. As with all AB cements, the dentist should take care to insure that at least 1 mm of sound dentin surrounds the pulp for any preparation, avoid desiccation and bacterial contamination, and use proper cementation technique to optimize pulpal health [3].

Definitive luting agents—contemporary

Resin-modified glass-ionomer (resin-modified glass polyalkenoate)

In the 1980s, with the desire to improve toughness and resistance to dissolution, water-soluble polymers or polymerizable resins were added to conventional glass-ionomers to create a new category of luting agent called resin-modified glass-ionomer cement (RMGI) [17,22]. In the original material, part of the water component of glass polyalkenoate cement was replaced with a water-hydroxymethyl methacrylate (HMMA) mixture, plus an initiator/activator for the added resin. Newer systems are more complex, and include other dimethacrylates such as ethylene glycol dimethacrylate and glycidylmethacrylate and Bisphenol A epoxy (Bis-GMA), as well as various chemicals to initiate and control the resin polymerization [8].

Resin-modified glass-ionomer is a dual-cure hybrid, because setting occurs by a combination of the long-term, complex acid-base reaction typical of glass-ionomer cement and chemical or light-initiated polymerization of the added resin. The acid-base reaction is slow because of reduced water content, so that initial hardening results from polymerization of the resin. The acid-base reaction continues to develop a polysalt hydrolgel matrix, which hardens and strengthens the existing polymer matrix [8]. If too little water is present or if the resin percentage is too high, only the polymerization reaction occurs, and the material acts like a filled, reinforced resin and is called a "compomer" (discussed below). Mount [17] commented that materials of this nature are often marketed so as to be confusing to the profession.

RMGI is less susceptible to early erosion during setting, less soluble, and has higher compressive and tensile strengths than unmodified glass-ionomer luting cement. Film thickness and adhesion to tooth structure are similar [16]. Fluoride release occurs to enhance cariostatic potential, but the amount varies by product [3]. Most RMGI cements come encapsulated, which simplifies mixing, but cost can be a factor because the unit dose price can be up to 35 times that of zinc phosphate [4]. To take advantage of the resin content in RMGI, the use of various adhesive systems has been tried to improve bond strength to tooth, but these have yielded mixed results [23]. Removal of the smear layer before cementation by acid etching is not typically needed for adequate retention, and may not be advisable because of a higher risk of post-cementation sensitivity [22]. RMGI is not without its' problems. Clinically, mixing and restoration placement is similar to encapsulated conventional glass-ionomer luting cement, with the ready-to-use material having a glossy surface, and firm finger pressure being used to facilitate complete seating of the restoration. As happens for conventional glass-ionomer, a snap set occurs, yet compared with unmodified glass-ionomer, the bulk is very hard, and removal can become a significant problem. If one waits over several minutes to remove the excess, or if one is cementing in the posterior areas of the mouth where embrasures are small and tooth contacts large, proper removal of cement can be extremely difficult to accomplish without damage to tissues, which would expose the early cement margin to blood and saliva, greatly reducing bond strength and accelerating erosion [22,24]. A dilemma results in that removal of excess must occur right after the initial set, which may pull unset material from under the restoration margin.

As for conventional glass-ionomer, RMGI is susceptible to dehydration shrinkage, which may occur up to several months post-insertion, creating stress fractures at the exposed cement tooth-restoration interface [16]. A petroleum jelly covering, as mentioned previously, may help limit the problem. Overall curing shrinkage is greater for RMGI, plus the hydrophilic nature of the added resin results in a varied degree of long-term water sorption, leading to volumetric expansion. Together these factors have caused concerns about the long-term dimensional stability and the constancy of the physical properties of RMGI [22,25]. RMGI should not be used for all-ceramic crowns or dowel (post) cementation, where such expansion could prove deleterious [16,22].

Compomers

The addition of resin to conventional glass-ionomer lead to the evolution of a diverse group of potential luting materials, which now represent a broad spectrum of compositions ranging from conventional glass-ionomer to composite resin. Depending on where a material lies on the spectrum determines the setting reactions and physical properties [17,24]. The compomers, also known as polyacid-modified composite resins, appeared in the late1990s [26], and were described as being a combination of composite resin (comp) and glass-ionomer (omer), offering the advantages of both [17]. Compomers are really anhydrous resins that contain ion-leachable glass as part of the filler, and dehydrated polyalkenoic acid. The original assumption was that continual water uptake by the resin would lead to an eventual AB cement reaction [17,24].

The physical behavior of compomers is more like composite resins than glass-ionomer, with higher compressive and flexural strengths than

RMGI, but inferior to unmodified composite [26]. Little if any tooth adhesion occurs without a resin bonding agent, and fluoride release is very limited [17]. Fluoride recharge occurs, but is less than that of conventional glass-ionomer [27].

Resin

Methyl methacrylate-based resin cement has been available since 1952 for cementation of indirect restorations [9]. Reformulations and improvements over the last 20 years, driven by a demand for all-ceramic and bonded restorations, have increased resin's popularity [2]. Resin cements are methyl methacrylate-, Bis-GMA dimethacrylate-, or urethane dimethacrylate-based, with fillers of colloidal silica or barium glass 20% to 80% by weight [10]. They are available as powder/liquid, encapsulated, or paste/paste systems, and may be auto-, dual-, or light-cured to form the polymer matrix.

Resin bonding to enamel is by micromechanical interlocking into an acid-etched surface. Bonding to dentin is also micromechanical, but is much more complex, usually requiring multiple steps that include removal of the smear layer and surface demineralization, then application of an unfilled resin bonding agent or primer, to which the resin chemically bonds. The practice of total etching, which frequently resulted in postoperative sensitivity, has been deemed not necessary and has been replaced by less invasive self-etching methods [28]. Residual eugenol from provisional cement can interfere with the setting reaction of the bonding agent, so non-eugenol provisional cement is recommended when resin will be used for the definitive restoration [24]. Polymerization shrinkage of the luting resin (depending on the bulk) may be significant enough to generate stresses that can form small gaps at the cement/tooth interface [16].

Many new resin luting systems have recently appeared that reduce luting procedures by including the use of self-etch adhesives. Multipurpose encapsulated resin cements that have a self-etch primer built-in (ie, Unicem by 3M ESPE; Maxcem by Kerr, Orange, California; and others) have gained extreme popularity, even though they lack long-term performance data [29].

How a resin cement is cured and the adhesive system used have been shown to have an impact on the quality of bond to hard dental tissues (ie, not all resin cement systems are equal in strength or performance) [30]. Light-cured resin cements are cured more completely after initial placement, whereas auto- and dual-cured resins slowly gain strength. Recent load fatigue testing (which is considered to be more clinically relevant than traditional tests) of gold crowns luted with several auto-curing resins demonstrated no superior performance compared with zinc phosphate [31].

Resin cements chemically bond to etched, silane-treated porcelain [16]. In general, resin cements are considered the best choice for luting all-ceramic restorations, based on multiple laboratory and clinical studies looking at fracture resistance and sealing. It has been postulated that resin cement bonded to conditioned tooth on one side and etched/silane coated porcelain on the other helps diffuse stresses across the tooth [32]. Finite element analysis has indicated that resin shrinkage during curing places bonded ceramic under compressive stress that helps protect the ceramic from tensile forces [33].

Many newer all-ceramic systems use milled zirconium or alumina substructures for single crowns and fixed partial dentures that cannot be internally etched, and have sufficient strengths to be luted with conventional cements. Even so, those restorations do not fit as well as metal or metalceramics, and may benefit from the high compressive strength and low solubility of a resin luting agent.

Because of the diversity of products and their ingredients, physical properties for resin cements vary, but certain generalizations can be made [10]. Compressive and tensile strength, toughness, and resilience of resin cement equal or exceed those of other luting agents; solubility is exceptionally low; and esthetic qualities are good, with color choices available. Conversely, resin luting cement offers no fluoride release or uptake; film thickness may be relatively high; pulpal compatibility may be an issue, especially for deep preparations; removal of a restoration may require total destruction; and a low elastic modulus (stiffness) may be a detriment for supporting brittle multi-unit all-ceramic prostheses [3,10,17,25,34]. Resins are more technique- sensitive and expensive per unit dose than conventional cements (up to 175 times the cost of zinc phosphate) [4], and as for RMGI, cleanup of excess cement can be very difficult.

Using resin cement for luting prefabricated and cast metal dowels placed in endodontically treated teeth has become popular because of its high-tensile strength and dentin-bonding ability. A resin luting agent would probably be the best choice for a prefabricated dowel that would be incorporated into a resin core to take advantage of exposed dowel cement bonding to core material. A recent study comparing cast metal dowel retention using zinc phosphate and an adhesive resin cement (Panavia F2.0, Kuraray Medical, Tokyo, Japan) found that the former provided greater tensile bond strength values [35]. Zinc phosphate may be a better choice than resin for luting a cast dowel core or prefabricated dowel to be placed in amalgam buildup, because of its longer working time and lower viscosity, which would facilitate complete seating of the dowel and high early strength, allowing quicker preparation, and lower cost.

Adhesive resin

In the early 1980s, conventional Bis-GMA resin cement was modified by adding a phosphate ester to the monomer component, introducing to dentistry a unique group of resin luting agents that have a degree of chemical bonding as well as a micromechanical bonding to tooth structure and base metal alloys. The first product marketed, Panavia (Morita, Osaka, Japan), contained the bifunctional adhesive monomer 10-methacryloyloxydecyl dihydrogen phosphate (MDP), and was a powder/liquid system. Bond strength to etched base metal greatly exceeded that to tooth, and Panavia quickly became the luting agent of choice for resin retained fixed partial dentures. Testing as a luting agent for single unit gold crowns indicated that Panavia gave higher retentive values than either zinc phosphate or conventional resin cement, even though retention to the metal was only micromechanical [36].

In 1994, Panavia was modified to include a dentin/enamel primer containing hydroxethyl methacrylate (HEMA), N-methacryloyl 5-aminosalicylic acid, and MDP, intended to improve bond strength to dentin. Under a new name, Panavia 21 (Morita, Osaka, Japan), it was marketed as a two-paste system that offered three shades: tooth colored (TC, translucent), white (EX, semitranslucent), and opaque (OP). Polymerization required exclusion of oxygen, and a covering gel was provided [37]. The current product, Panavia F, is a two-paste system that is dual-cured, self-etching, and self-adhesive, plus fluoride-releasing. Bonding to base metal is good, and is optimized by air abrasion with alumina oxide, followed by use of pyrolized silane [12]. Noble metal bonding is fair after tin plating or abrasion, and improved with the use of a newly introduced metal primer [38,39].

Before the introduction of Panavia, Bis-GMA composite was modified by decreasing filler and adding 3% 2hydroxy-3b-napthoxypropyl methacrylate in methyl methacrylate with 4-methacryloyloxyethyl trimellitate anhydride (4-META) and tri-n-butyl borane, and marketed as C & B Metabond (Parkell, Farmingdale, New York). C & B Metabond has physical characteristics similar to other resin cements, but also has an extremely high tensile strength, which is useful for providing retention in restorative situations where less than optimal conditions exist. It is a powder/liquid auto-curing system, and may be used for resin-bonded prostheses. The set cement has a chalky appearance, no inorganic fillers, and is not radiopaque [35].

Panavia and C & B Metabond represent several available unique adhesive resin luting agents of various compositions that can help provide adequate retention for crowns and prostheses where less than ideal retention exists [37]. In general, these materials are expensive, very technique-sensitive, difficult to clean up when set, and do not have an exceptionally long shelf life.

Cement considerations for implant-supported crowns

Much of what we know and how we think about cements has been learned from their use with teeth. Luting considerations for cemented implant-supported crowns differ slightly, and depend on the type of prosthesis and long-term goals. Basic requirements (mechanical, biological, and handling requirements previously discussed) must be met by the luting agent, but some properties (ie, fluoride release, bonding to tooth, and so on) are not needed for these restorations.

Studies have shown that cement-retained, implant-supported crowns luted with zinc phosphate and glass ionomer do not have the same quality of marginal fit as do their screw- retained counterparts [40]. Both have clinically acceptable strength qualities, but may have solubility issues if exposed to oral fluids too early. It may be difficult to achieve or maintain a dry cementing environment for crowns placed on deep subgingival abutment margins, which often occur in esthetic areas [41]. Therefore, a resin or RMGI cement of relatively low solubility may seem to be the better choice.

Removal of excess material after cementation can be a major concern. Sadan and colleagues [41] commented, "The biggest challenge of a cemented (implant-supported) restoration is the complexity in clinical delivery... and cleaning the cement excess." Rapid onset complications associated with excess cement left around crowns on implants have been documented, and a 1-week post-cementation follow-up is recommended to examine peri-implant tissues for problems [42]. Agar and coworkers [43] compared zinc phosphate, glass ionomer, and resin cements for ease of removal from titanium abutments and accompanying instrument damage, and found that zinc phosphate was the easiest to remove and resin the most difficult. They also recommended plastic scalers for removal of excess material, to avoid metal scratches. Ease of excess removal indicates that conventional cement might be the best choice for luting a cemented implant-supported crown.

The last major concern to be discussed is that of cement strength. Is the luted implant-supported crown or prosthesis intended to be retrievable (ie, is intentional removal at some later time desirable)? If so, then the natural inclination would be to use provisional cement. Akca and colleagues [44] observed that single-unit, cemented, implant-supported crowns luted with provisional cements necessitate frequent recementation, and thus recommended that temporary cements be used only for multiple-unit implant-supported prostheses. Recementation can be very difficult, especially if surrounding tissues quickly collapse around the abutment [41].

Some feel that the cemented restoration should be retrievable, in order to facilitate tightening of the abutment screw. Sadan [45] pointed out that abutment screw loosening is not a given occurrence, and is indicative of failure to follow proper clinical and laboratory protocols. Single crowns (especially all-ceramic) cannot simply be tapped off, and retrieval may result in total destruction of the restoration. He commented, "The clinician should use the strongest cement available and, whenever possible, achieve a bond between the restoration and the abutment" [45]. According to in-vitro studies, resin cements provide the highest retentive strength for luted implant components or implant-supported crowns. Other luting materials vary in rank order of retentiveness, and their behavior may be different than when natural teeth serve as abutments [46,47].

Fatigue failure?

Early in this discussion it was stated that a definitive luting agent's primary requirement is to hold an indirect restoration in place for an indefinite period of time, and maintain a seal between restoration and tooth. Measurements made for comparison of cements by characteristics such as compressive and tensile strengths, retention, and so on, are significant, but have been done under static, unidirectional testing, and may only represent the early state of a newly cemented restoration.

In recent years, it has been recognized that during function, luted restorations undergo repetitive dynamic loading that might lead to cement failure through fatigue (breaking or fracturing of the material caused by cyclic loading below the yield limit [1]) [48]. In theory, fatigue cement fracture clinically leads to fluid microleakage with bacterial ingress, which can cascade to eventual recurrent caries or loss of retention to the point of restoration failure [31]. The empirical observation that many well-designed and properly cemented indirect restorations do not eventually fail because of cement fatigue means that many factors (ie, abutment taper and resistance form [49], preparation height and diameter [50], and the like) influence the stresses placed on luting cement. Even so, cement fatigue failure probably does occur in many instances, and dynamic load fatigue testing (along with thermal cycling) may help understand long-term clinical performance and aid in comparison of these materials [31].

Summary

The pros and cons of definitive luting cements have been reviewed, and indeed, none are ideal. Selection of luting agent to be used for a given restoration should not be an arbitrary choice. It must be based on a basic knowledge of the materials available, the type of restoration to be placed, and the requirements defined by the patient (ie, high caries index, all-ceramic restoration, and so on). Newer restorative options have altered the priority of requirements of luting cement and the marketplace has responded. Claims by manufacturers of "one universal cement" applicable for all indirect restorations may be partly true, in that one luting agent (resin) can be used in all situations and for all patients. But is it the best choice every time? Many clinical situations will continue to present where conventional luting cements would best serve the need. Older, tried and tested materials must not be ignored or pushed aside, yet the prudent clinician should diligently keep up with new technology.

References

[1] The Academy of Prosthodontics. The glossary of prosthodontic terms. J Prosthet Dent 2005; 94(1):21–38.

[2] Clinical Research Associates. CRA Newsletter, Clinicians' guide to dental products & techniques 2004;28(10):1–2.

[3] Rosenstiel SF, Land MF, Crispin BJ. Dental luting agents: a review of the current literature. J Prosthet Dent 1998;80(3):280–301.

[4] de la Macorra JC, Pradies G. Conventional and adhesive luting cements. Clin Oral Investig 2002;6:198–204.

[5] Smith DC. Dental cements current status and future prospects. Dent Clin North Am 1983; 6(3):763–93.

[6] Donovan TE, Cho GC. Contemporary evaluation of dental cements. Compend Contin Educ Dent 1999;20(3):197–219.

[7] Craig RG, Powers JM. Restorative dental materials. 11th edition. St Louis: Mosby; 2002. p. 594–634.

[8] Wilson AD, Nicholson JW. Acid-base cements, their biomedical and industrial applications. New York: Cambridge University Press; 1993. p. 1–383.

[9] Craig RG. Restorative dental materials. 8th edition. St Louis: Mosby; 1989. p. 189–225.

[10] O'Brien W. Dental materials and their selection. 3rd edition. Chicago: Quintessence; 2002. p. 133–55.

[11] Shillingburg HT, Hobo S, Whitsett LD, et al. Fundamentals of fixed prosthodontics. 3rd edition. Chicago: Quintessence; 1997. p. 400–12, 538.

[12] Goodacre CJ, Campagni WV, Aquilino SA. Tooth preparations for complete crowns: an art form based on scientific principals. J Prosthet Dent 2001;85(4):363–76.

[13] Pameijer CH, Stanley HR, Ecker G. Biocompatibility of a glass ionomer luting agent. Part II: Crown cementation. Am J Dent 1991;4(3):134–41.

[14] Johnson GH, Hazelton LR, Bales DJ, et al. The effect of a resin-based sealer on crown retention for three types of cement. J Prosthet Dent 2004;91(5):428–35.

[15] Smith DC. A new dental cement. Br Dent J 1968;125:381–4.

[16] Diaz-Arnold AM, Vargas MA, Haselton DR. Current status of luting agents for fixed prosthodontics. J Prosthet Dent 1999;81(2):135–41.

[17] Mount GJ. An atlas of glass-ionomer cements, a clinicians guide. 3rd edition. New York: Martin Duntiz; 2002. p. 1–73.

[18] Prentice LH, Tyas MJ, Burrow MF. The effect of mixing time on the handling and compressive strength of encapsulated glass-ionomer cement. Dent Mater 2005;21(8): 704–8.

[19] Curtis SR, Richards MW, Meiers JC. Early erosion of glass-ionomer at crown margins. Int J Prosthodont 1993;6(6):553–7.

[20] Ogimoto T, Ogawa T. Simple and sure protection of crown margins from moisture in cementation. J Prosthet Dent 1997;78(2):225.

[21] Gandolfi MG, Chersoni S, Acquaviva GL, et al. Fluoride release and adsorption at different pH from glass-ionomer cements. Dent Mater 2006;22(5):441–9.

[22] Davidson CL, Mjor IA. Advances in glass-ionomer cements. Chicago: Quintessence; 1999. p. 41–3, 160–6, 247–50.

[23] Wang L, Sakai VT, Kawai ES, et al. Effects of adhesive systems associated with resin-modified glass-ionomer cements. J Oral Rehabil 2006;33(2):110–6.

[24] Albers HF. Tooth-colored restoratives, principles and techniques. 9th edition. London: BC Decker; 2002. p. 43–127.

[25] Platt JA. Resin cements: into the 21st century. Compend Contin Educ Dent 1999;20(12): 1172–81.

[26] Meyer JM, Cattani-Lorente MA, Dupuis V. Compomers—between glass-ionomer cements and composites. Biomaterials 1998;19(6):529–39.

[27] Cildir SK, Sandalli N. Fluoride release/uptake of glass-ionomer cements and polyacid-modified composite resins. Dent Mater J 2005;24(1):92–7.

[28] Christensen GJ. Has the "total-etch" concept disappeared? J Am Dent Assoc 2006;137(6): 817–20.

[29] Clinical Research Associates. CRA newsletter, Special product report—product use survey. 2005;29(10):1–2.

[30] Piwowarczyk A, Bender R, Ottl P, et al. Long-term bond between dual-polymerizing cementing agents and human hard dental tissue. Dent Mater 2006; (Epub ahead of print).

[31] Uy JN, Lian JN, Nichols JI, et al. Load-fatigue performance of gold crowns luted with resin cements. J Prosthet Dent 2006;95(4):315–22.

[32] Burke FJ, Fleming GJ, Nathanson D, et al. Are adhesive technologies needed to support ceramics? An assessment of the current evidence. J Adhes Dent 2002;4(1):7–22.

[33] Magne P, Versluis A, Douglas WH. Effect of luting composite shrinkage and thermal loads on the stress distribution in porcelain laminate veneers. J Prosthet Dent 1999;81(3):335–43.

[34] Zhen CL, White S. Mechanical properties of dental luting cements. J Prosthet Dent 1999; 81(5):597–609.

[35] Ertugrul HZ, Ismail YH. An in-vitro comparison of cast metal dowel retention using various luting agents and tensile loading. J Prosthet Dent 2005;93(5):446–52.

[36] Tjan AHL, Tao L. Seating and retention of complete crowns with a new adhesive resin cement. J Prosthet Dent 1992;67(4):478–83.

[37] McComb D. Adhesive luting cements—classes, criteria, and usage. Compend Contin Educ Dent 1996;17(8):759–73.

[38] Petrie CS, Eick JD, Williams K, et al. A comparison of three alloy surface treatments for resin-bonded prostheses. J Prosthodont 2001;10(4):217–33.

[39] Zidan O, Ferfuson GC. The retention of complete crowns prepared with three different tapers and luted with four different cements. J Prosthet Dent 2003;89(6):565–71.

[40] Keith SE, Miller BH, Woody RD, et al. Marginal discrepancy of screw-retained and cemented metal-ceramic crowns on implant abutments. Int J Oral Maxillofac Implants 1999;14(3):369–78.

[41] Sadan A, Blatz MB, Bellerino M, et al. Prosthetic design considerations for anterior single-implant restorations. Inside Dentistry 2006;2(6):30–5.

[42] Pauletto N, Lahiffe BJ, Walton JN. Complications associated with excess cement around crowns on osseointegrated implants: a clinical report. Int J Oral Maxillofac Implants 1999;14(6):865–8.

[43] Agar JR, Cameron SM, Hughbanks JC, et al. Cement removal from restorations luted to titanium abutments with simulated subgingival margins. J Prosthet Dent 1997;78(1):43–7.

[44] Akca K, Iplikcioglu H, Cehreli MC. Comparison of uniaxial resistance forces of cements used with implant-supported crowns. Int J Oral Maxillofac Implants 2002;17(4):536–42.

[45] Sada A. Cement considerations for implant-supported restorations. Pract Periodontics Aesthet Dent 2000;12(4):356.

[46] Mansour A, Ercoli C, Graser G, et al. Comparative evaluation of casting retention using the ITI solid abutment with six cements. Clin Oral Implants Res 2002;13(4):343–8.

[47] Squier RS, Agar JR, Duncan JP, et al. Retentiveness of dental cements used with metallic implant components. Int J Oral Maxillofac Implants 2001;16(6):793–8.

[48] Wiskott HW, Nicholls JI, Belser UC. Stress fatigue: basic principles and prosthodontic implications. Int J Prosthodont 1995;8(2):105–16.

[49] Wiskott HW, Nicholls JI, Belser UC. The relationship between abutment taper and resistance of cemented crowns to dynamic loading. Int J Prosthodont 1996;9(2):117–39.

[50] Wiskott HW, Nicholls JI, Belser UC. The effect of tooth preparation height and diameter on the resistance of complete crowns to fatigue loading. Int J Prosthodont 1997;10(3):207–15.

ELSEVIER
SAUNDERS

Dent Clin N Am 51 (2007) 659–675

THE DENTAL
CLINICS
OF NORTH AMERICA

Direct Composite Restorative Materials

Aaron D. Puckett, PhD[a],*, James G. Fitchie, DMD[a],
Pia Chaterjee Kirk, DDS[a], Jefferson Gamblin, BS[b]

[a]Care Planning and Restorative Sciences, University of Mississippi Medical Center,
School of Dentistry, 2500 North State Street, Jackson, MS 39216, USA
[b]University of Mississippi Medical Center, School of Dentistry, 2500 North State Street,
Jackson, MS 39216, USA

A generalized definition of a composite is a multiphase material that exhibits the properties of both phases where the phases are complimentary, resulting in a material with enhanced properties [1]. The materials discussed in this article are composites by definition that are used as direct esthetic restorative materials.

The first tooth-colored composite was silicate cement, which was introduced in 1870s. This composite formulation was based on alumino-fluro-silicate glasses and phosphoric acid. The dispersed phase was residual glass particles, and the matrix phase was the aluminum phosphate salt formed from the partial acid dissolution of the glass particles; however, these were brittle, required mechanical retention, and had an average longevity of only a few years [2].

The first polymeric tooth-colored composite used in dentistry was based on poly(methylmethacrylate). This material was developed in the 1940s, and consisted of a poly(methylmethacrylate) powder, methyl methacrylate monomer, benzoyl peroxide, and n,n-dimethlyparatoluidine. These materials could be classified as composites, because upon mixing, the polymer powder formed a dispersed phase and the monomer polymerized to form the continuous phase. The polymerization was initiated at room temperature, using the redox initiator combination of benzoyl peroxide and n,n-dimethlyparatoluidine. Although these materials were initially esthetic, they were plagued with a variety of problems, including poor color stability, high polymerization shrinkage, a lack of bonding to tooth structure, and a large coefficient of thermal expansion (CTE) [2].

---

* Corresponding author.
  E-mail address: apuckett@sod.umsmed.edu (A.D. Puckett).

0011-8532/07/$ - see front matter © 2007 Elsevier Inc. All rights reserved.
doi:10.1016/j.cden.2007.04.003 *dental.theclinics.com*

The first polymer matrix composite incorporating silica fillers was introduced in the 1950s. These composites had improved mechanical properties and good esthetics; they did not bond to tooth structure, and still exhibited significant polymerization shrinkage. In addition, there was no significant bonding between the silica particles and the polymer matrix. Consequently, these composites did not have good wear resistance clinically, because the filler particles were easily dislodged [3]. New improved formulations incorporated a coupling agent such as γ-methacryloxpropyl-trimethoxy silane or vinyl triethoxysilane. The coupling agent provided a method to covalently bond the filler particles to the resin matrix. The resulting composite exhibited improved mechanical properties and wear resistance; however, the polymerization shrinkage and lack of bonding to tooth structure limited the clinical success of these formulations.

One way to address the polymerization shrinkage problem is to use high molecular weight monomers. In 1962 Bowen [4,5], while at the National Bureau of Standards, synthesized an acrylated epoxy using glycidylmethacrylate and Bisphenol A epoxy for use as a matrix for dental composite. The resulting monomer, called Bis-GMA or Bowen's resin, possessed the viscosity of honey, and therefore limited the amount of filler particles that could be incorporated. Subsequent experiments incorporated triethylene glycol dimethacrylate (TEGDMA) as a diluent to reduce the viscosity. This monomer combination worked well, and has become one of the most widely used matrix monomer combinations for dental composites to date. The structures of Bis-GMA and TEGDMA are shown in Figs. 1 and 2, respectively. Both of these monomers contain two reactive double bonds, and when polymerized, form covalent bonds between the polymer chains known as cross-links. Cross-linking improved the properties of the matrix phase, and the composite produced had improved mechanical and physical properties [3]. Additional composite formulations have been prepared using various diluent monomers such as methyl methacrylate (MMA) and ethylene glycol dimethacrylate (EGDMA), and an additional high molecular weight monomer based on a urethane dimethacrylate (UDMA). The chemical structure for UDMA is illustrated in Fig. 3.

Additional monomers based on poly-acid modified acrylates have been used to formulate composites called compomers. The fillers used in compomers are silicate-based glasses and sodium fluoride. They are polymerized using free radical chemistry initiated by photoactive species or redox initiator systems. These materials were designed to have the handling

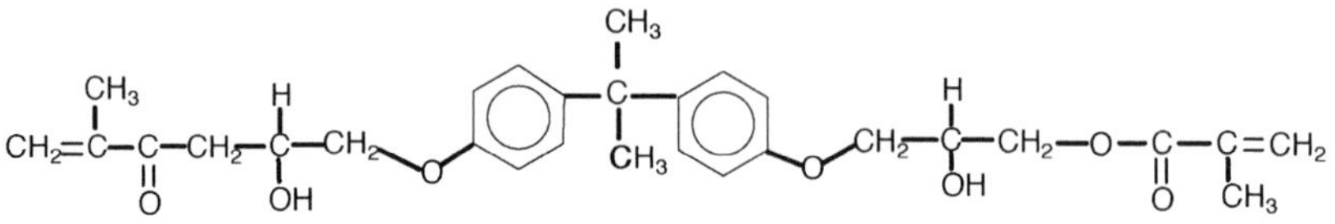

Fig. 1. Chemical structure of Bis-GMA.

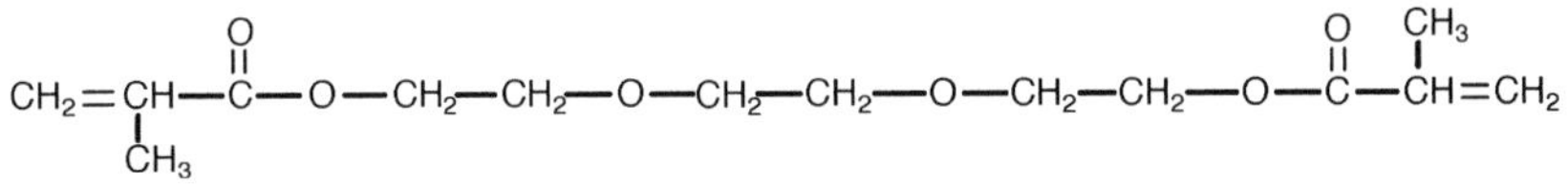

$$CH_2=CH-\overset{\overset{\displaystyle O}{\|}}{\underset{\underset{\displaystyle CH_3}{|}}{C}}-O-CH_2-CH_2-O-CH_2-CH_2-O-CH_2-CH_2-O-\overset{\overset{\displaystyle O}{\|}}{C}-\overset{\overset{\displaystyle CH_3}{|}}{CH}=CH_2$$

Fig. 2. Chemical structure of triethylene glycol dimethacrylate.

properties of a traditional resin composite and the fluoride-releasing properties of a glass ionomer. Because of the hydrophilic nature of the resins,
compomers actually absorb fluid from the oral environment, causing an
expansion of the composite that offsets a portion of the polymerization
shrinkage which occurs during setting. Compomers do not have the
mechanical properties of more traditional composites, or the amount of
fluoride release of glass ionomers, but have been used successfully as a direct
restorative resin in some applications [2].

Composite fillers

The reinforcing phase in direct dental restoratives is based on glass or
ceramic particles. Incorporation of these inorganic particles imparts
improved strength and wear properties, decreased CTE, and reduced polymerization shrinkage. In addition, incorporation of heavy metals into the
filler provide radiopacity. The initial composite fillers were limited in size
because of the limited ability to grind and sieve quartz, glass, borosilicate,
or ceramic particles. The particle size range was from 0.1 to 100 μm. Smaller
particles have been prepared through hydrolysis or precipitation to produce
what is termed fumed or pyrolitic silica. The particle sizes obtained from this
process range from 0.06 to 0.1 μm [6].

The most recent process to form particles is through sol-gel chemistry,
which uses silicate precursors that are polymerized to form particles ranging
from nm to μm dimensions [7]. This sol-gel process can be used to form almost mono dispersed particle sizes, which can be a significant advantage
because different particle sizes can be produced and blended to optimize
the packing efficiency and filler loading of the composite. In addition, the
ability to produce submicron size particles allows the production of nanocomposites in which the particles approach the size of the polymer matrix
molecules. Theoretically, nanocomposites have the potential to exhibit
excellent mechanical and physical properties at higher filler loadings [8].

Composite resin chemistry

To reduce polymerization shrinkage and increase mechanical and physical properties requires the use of high molecular weight monomers that have

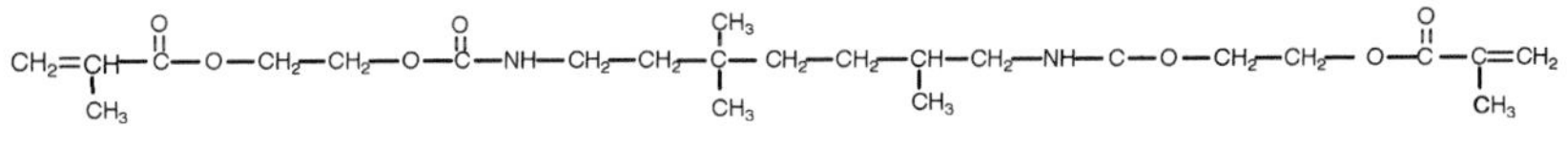

$$CH_2=CH-\overset{\overset{\displaystyle O}{\|}}{\underset{\underset{\displaystyle CH_3}{|}}{C}}-O-CH_2-CH_2-O-\overset{\overset{\displaystyle O}{\|}}{C}-NH-CH_2-CH_2-\overset{\overset{\displaystyle CH_3}{|}}{\underset{\underset{\displaystyle CH_3}{|}}{C}}-CH_2-CH_2-\overset{\overset{\displaystyle}{|}}{\underset{\underset{\displaystyle CH_3}{|}}{CH}}-CH_2-NH-C-O-CH_2-CH_2-O-\overset{\overset{\displaystyle O}{\|}}{C}-\overset{\overset{\displaystyle}{|}}{\underset{\underset{\displaystyle CH_3}{|}}{C}}=CH_2$$

Fig. 3. Chemical structure of urethane dimethacrylate (UDMA).

the ability to cross-link. The high molecular weight reduces the volume change during polymerization. Cross-linking forms covalent bonds between the polymer chains, resulting in a dramatic increase in modulus and reduction in solubility [3]. Bowen's resin is the reaction product between Bisphenol A and glycidyl dimethacrylate. The chemical name is 2,2-bis[4-(2 hydroxy-3 methacryloxy proproxy)-phenyl]-propane, but it is commonly referred to as Bis-GMA. This long-chain monomer is multifunctional, having two methacrylate groups that allow it to cross-link during polymerization; however, because of its large size, Bis-GMA is highly viscous, and limits the ability to formulate composites having high filler loadings. Consequently, a lower molecular weight monomer such triethylene glycol dimethacrylate (TEGDMA) or EDMA is added to reduce the viscosity and allow increased filler loadings to be used. These monomers are also multifunctional and increase the number of cross-linking reactions during setting of resin matrix. These lower viscosity monomers may comprise 10% to 50% of a composite's composition.

Although these monomers allow increased filler concentrations, their incorporation can lead to greater polymerization shrinkage. In addition, these monomers can produce composites with increased flexibility and decreased abrasion resistance. It has been suggested that these low molecular weight monomers increase the time before gelation of the matrix occurs, and subsequently reduce marginal polymerization contraction stress [3,9]. Consequently, incorporation of these monomers can have both positive and negative effects on the composite's properties.

One of the most significant problems with current monomers used for direct composite restorative materials is the shrinkage that occurs during polymerization. Currently, all commercial dental composites are based on vinyl monomers polymerized using free radical initiators. Conversion of these monomers results in a decrease in distance between the molecules, from a Van der Waals gap to the distance of a covalent bond. Although this distance is very small for a single monomer, the distance change over a long polymer chain is significant. Inclusion of filler reduces the volume of resin and its volume change, but the amount of filler incorporation is approaching the maximum theoretical packing fraction of 74 volume % for close-packed structures [3]. The amount of shrinkage is controlled by the volume of resin, its composition, and the degree of conversion. Current commercial dental composites have a volumetric shrinkage ranging from 1.6 to 8 volume % [3,10]. The contraction stress developed at the margin of the restoration can be sufficient to overcome the bond strength of the bonding system, resulting in a contraction gap [11,12]. The contraction gap can lead to microleakage and all its associated problems (eg, secondary caries and pain).

In a recent study, the contraction stress was measured to range from 3.3 to 23.5 Mpa [9]. During polymerization at room temperature, the resin matrix gels, and the polymer formed is below its glass transition temperature (Tg). Therefore, the amount of flow available to the polymer matrix to relieve the contraction stress during polymerization is limited. Low molecular weight diluent resins can provide more flow, but have the potential to reduce the mechanical properties of the matrix. The relationship between contraction stress and composite composition is complex, but Kleverlann and Feilzer [9] did find correlations between volumetric shrinkage and contraction stress that suggest that lower amounts of shrinkage in current highly filled composites actually result in higher contraction stress. This surprising result may be related to the ability of formulations that contain higher concentrations of low molecular weight monomers being able to reduce contraction stress by molecular relaxations and flow.

One approach to reduce polymerization shrinkage and contraction stress is through the development of low-shrinkage or expanding monomer systems. These resin systems are based on ring-opening polymerization reactions that do not shrink to the extent of conventional vinyl polymerization resins. Monomers based on spiro-ortho carbonate have been prepared and evaluated in composite formulations. Although the composites formulated using these monomers did show less polymerization shrinkage, the property improvements were only incremental, and probably not significant enough to be realized clinically [13,14].

Eick and colleagues [15] have reported composite matrix resins based on cycloaliphatic expoxies. These resins are polymerized using photoactive cationic initiators. Although the resins show promise, they require further optimization before a commercial product can be produced.

Chen and colleagues [8] have developed another expoxy-based resin matrix, and prepared a composite that also incorporated nanofiller technology. The composite exhibited mechanical and physical properties that are comparable to commercial dental composites, and the strain measured during polymerization was significantly reduced. Based on these studies, commercialization of low-shrinkage monomers may be realized in the near future. The development of low-shrinkage or expanding monomers could be one of the most significant advances in direct dental restorative materials since their introduction.

One problem that has not been addressed is the large difference between the CTE of resin composites and tooth structure. The CTE of tooth structure ranges from 9 to 11 ppm/$°$C, compared with 28 to 50 ppm/$°$C for dental composite restoratives [16]. The differential expansion and contraction of composites cause additional stress at the margin of the restoration that contribute to fatigue failure of the bond between the composite and tooth structure. Currently the only way to lower the CTE of composites is to increase the filler loading.

Curing of dental composites

The majority of current dental composites are cured using visible light ranging from 450 to 475 nm. Light sources include quartz halogen, laser, plasma arc, and most recently, light emitting diodes (LED). The minimum energy required for adequate curing is 300 mW/cm^2. Newer lights have incorporated curing modes that step or ramp up the light intensity with time. These modes were added in an attempt to control the polymerization shrinkage and reduce the polymerization contraction stress. Although these lights have shown some promise, the clinical effectiveness of these controlled polymerization techniques is unknown. All of the lights used for curing composite increase the temperature of the composite to varying extents, which can actually increase the degree of conversion [17,18]; however, high-intensity light sources may cause sufficient temperature increases to result in damage to the pulp.

Composite classification: properties and applications

There has been a number of classification systems proposed to describe composite restoratives. One of the most often used classification systems is based upon filler particle size. As composite restoratives have evolved, the size of filler particles and their size distribution have been changed, in an attempt to achieve the best possible mechanical properties while maintaining esthetics. This discussion uses the following broad classifications: microfills, hybrids, packables, and compomers. In addition, subclassifications, including flowables, and nano- and microhybrids, are addressed. A summary of some of the characteristics for direct composite restoratives is given in Table 1.

Microfilled composites

Microfilled composites were introduced to the market from the late 1970s to the early 1980s. Microfilled composites were developed to provide the dental profession with a material that possessed outstanding polishability and esthetics. These composites incorporate particles ranging from 0.04 um

Table 1
Selected properties of direct composite restoratives

Composite classification	Filler content		Volume shrinkage (%)	Average particle size (μm)
	Weight %	Volume %		
Hybrid	74–87	57–72	1.6–4.7	0.2–3.0
Nanohybrid	72–87	58–71	2.0–3.4	0.4–0.9 (macro)
	—	—	—	0.015–0.05 (nano)
Microfills	35–80	20–59	2–3	0.04–0.75
Flowables	40–60	30–55	4–8	0.6–1.0
Compomers	59–77	43–61	2.6–3.4	0.7–0.8

Data from Rawls HR, Upshaw JE. Restorative resins. In: Anusavice KJ, editor. Phillip's science of dental materials. 11th edition. Philladelphia: WB Saunders; 2003. p. 399–441; and Miller MB. Reality: the information source for esthetic dentistry. Houston (TX): Reality Publishing Company; 2006.

to 0.4 um [3]. The early versions of microfilled resins were limited in the amount of filler that could be incorporated, because of the high surface area-to-volume ratio of the filler that caused large viscosity increases in the formulation. These composites only contained 35 to 67 weight % and 20 to 59 volume % glass fillers [3].

One way to increase the volume of small particles is through the use of prepolymerized particles. In this process, submicron-sized particles are mixed with monomers such a Bis-GMA and TEGDMA at elevated temperatures. The mixture is then cured at elevated temperature and pressure, using benzoyl peroxide as an initiator. After polymerization, the material is chilled and ground to form particles having a size range of 1 to 200 μm [6]. The prepolymerized particles allow higher filler loadings to be obtained with smaller particles; however, the prepolymerized particles cannot be bonded to the matrix phase using silane coupling agents. Interfacial bonding requires diffusion of the matrix monomers into the particles, with subsequent polymerization to provide micromechanical interlocks. Some investigators have suggested that the lack of interfacial bonding in these systems may contribute to failure [3,6].

Therefore microfilled composites have a lower elastic modulus and lower fracture strength than materials that contain higher concentrations of filler [19]. The prepolymerized particles allow the filler content to be maximized and polymerization shrinkage to be minimized, however, while making these composites highly polishable and possessing the ability to maintain a smooth surface during clinical wear [20]. Because of these properties, microfilled composite resins are indicated for Class V restorations, non–stress-bearing Class III restorations, and small Class I restorations. They are also indicated for direct composite resin veneers if the patient does not demonstrate any parafunctional habits, such as bruxism. Because of their lower fracture strength and potential for marginal breakdown, microfills are generally contraindicated for posterior load bearing restorations such as Class II and large Class I restorations [21]. The only exception is the microfill Heliomolar (Ivoclar-Vivadent), which may be used for posterior restorations because it has consistently shown excellent wear resistance and longevity compared with other resin composites [22]. The Classic examples of traditional microfilled composites in this category are Durafill (Heraeus Kulzer, Armonk, New York), Renamel microfill (Cosmedent, Chicago, Illinois), and Heliomolar.

A subclass of microfills that has recently been produced is referred to as flowable. These composites are lightly filled, and were developed to be used where limited access to the restoration made it difficult to adapt other composite types to the walls of the preparation. Flowable composites are composed of traditional composite resins with a filler loading reduced to 30 to 55 volume %, compared with 57 to 72 volume % for traditional hybrid resin composites [3,10]. The amount of fluidity or flowability varies significantly between various products. A study comparing the flowability of five materials found that Ultraseal XT Plus (Ultradent, South Jordan, Utah) had five times the flow of the least fluid, Aeliteflo, Bisco, Schaumburg, Illinois). Compared with a traditional hybrid, Aeliteflo exhibited the same amount of fluidity as Z100 (3M Espe, St. Paul, Minnesota) and one half of the fluidity as Prodigy (Kerr, Orange, California) [23]. Because of these wide differences in viscosities between materials, flowable composites vary considerably in polymerization shrinkage, stiffness, and other physical properties [24]. In addition, because of their decreased filler content and reduced physical properties, flowable composites are recommended for use in low-stress areas such as very small Class I occlusal restorations, similar to pit and fissure sealants or conservative composite restorations. Some clinicians prefer to use flowable composites for Class V carious lesions and abrasion/abfraction lesions because of their low modulus of elasticity and low viscosity. Theoretically, flowable composites will flex with the tooth in the areas of stress, because their elastic modulus is closer to that of the tooth structure. The flowable composites' relatively low elastic modulus could also reduce the stress transfer to tooth structure, and maintain the marginal seal in the Class V flexure situations. The use of flowable composites for the initial increment in the proximal box portion of a Class II restoration is at best controversial. One study found that a flowable composite layer is advantageous in reducing microleakage in a Class II restoration in vitro [25]. A study by Hilton and Quinn [26] found a nonsignificant trend toward reduced microleakage in thermocycled Class II restorations when a flowable composite was used in a thin layer under a nonflowable, resin-based composite. Other studies have failed to show differences in microleakage between restorations with and without a layer of flowable composite material [27,28]. The inconsistent findings associated with the use of flowable composites may be explained by the fact that even though they have a low elastic modulus, the contraction stresses produced by some of these materials could be sufficiently high to cause failure of the bond between composite layers, and at the composite/tooth interface when a flowable composite is used as a thin intermediate layer. A study by Braga and others [29] found that most of the flowable materials tested did not produce significant stress reduction when used under a nonflowable composite. It has been postulated that any favorable effects on limiting microleakage may be caused by improved adaptation to cavity walls and stress-absorbing properties outweighing the effects of increased polymerization shrinkage [30]. Despite the many controversies found in in vitro studies, many clinicians continue to use flowable composite as liners under traditional hybrid materials for the initial increment in the proximal boxes of Class II restorations.

Hybrid composites

The majority of resin composites in clinical use today are categorized in the general term of "hybrid composites." This broad category includes traditional hybrids, micro-, and nanohybrids. The "hybrid" moniker implies a resin composite blend containing submicron inorganic filler particles (.04 μm) and small particles (1 μm–4 μm). The combination of various sizes of filler particles corresponds to an improvement in physical properties as well as acceptable levels of polishability [31]. These improvements in wear resistance and fracture strength, along with good polishability, make hybrids the material of choice for Class III and Class IV restorations. In addition, practitioners have used these traditional hybrids in posterior load-bearing surfaces such as Class I and Class II restorations because of their improved strength and wear resistance.

Recent improvements in filler technology by manufacturers have allowed blends of both submicron particles (0.04 μm) and small particles (0.1 μm–1.0 μm) to be incorporated into a composite formulation. These materials are classified as micro-hybrid composites. The mixture of smaller particles distinguishes microhybrids from traditional hybrids and allows for a finer polish, along with improved handling. The desirable combination of strength and surface smoothness offers the clinician flexibility for use in posterior stress-bearing areas as well as anterior esthetic areas [32]. Although microhybrids offer superior strength, their polishability is not better than a traditional microfilled composite resin [33]. Examples of current microhybrid materials include Prodigy, Synergy (Coltene-Whaledent, Cuyahoga Falls, Ohio), Gradia Direct (GC America, Alsip, Illinois), Vitalescence (Ultradent), and Palfique Estelite (J. Morita USA, Irvine, California). The trend in the newer microhybrid materials is to maximize filler loading and minimize filler size [34]. The latest version of microfilled hybrids has used nanofiller technology to formulate what have been referred to as nanohybrid composite resins. Nanohybrids contain nanometer-sized filler particles (.005–.01 microns) throughout the resin matrix, in combination with a more conventional type filler technology. Nanohybrids may be classified as the first truly universal composite resin with handling properties and polishability of a microfilled composite, and the strength and wear resistance of a traditional hybrid [35]. These nanohybrids can be used in any situation similar to the microhybrids, with possibly a slight improvement in polishability because of the smaller particle size. Examples of nanofilled resin-based composites are Filtex Supreme (3M Espe) and Premise (Kerr, Orange, California).

Packable composites

Packable or condensable composites were developed to provide a composite that handled more like amalgam. This marketing ploy by dental product manufacturers was an attempt to increase the use of composites by older dentists who were not trained in their use in dental school, and younger dentists who were looking for a more user-friendly material. Packable composites have a higher viscosity and are less "sticky" than other composite restoratives. The viscosity increase is obtained through changes in the particle size distribution and incorporation of fibers [3]. These composites were introduced to the market as amalgam substitutes, as practitioners searched for the ideal esthetic material with handling properties similar to amalgam. Another desire was to find a material that would establish adequate proximal contacts more easily than traditional hybrid composites. Claims of improved handling properties and better adaptation to the matrix band in Class II restorations have piqued the interest of many clinicians. A study by Brackett and Covey [36] compared the condensability of spherical amalgam, admixed amalgam, conventional hybrid composite resins, and condensable composite resins. They found that the compressive forces for two condensable composites were significantly less than all four amalgams. As a result, the dental profession has referred to these materials as "packable composites" instead of "condensable," because of their greater viscosity and decreased stickiness compared with conventional hybrid composites. When initially placed, these materials were more viscous than traditional hybrid composites; however, after placement the viscosity decreased as the temperature of the material equilibrated with the temperature of the oral cavity [37]. Although the "packable composites" showed improved handling properties for restoring Class I and II preparations, they have not fully solved the problem of achieving adequate interproximal contacts. Some clinicians still prefer their stiffer consistency; however, the physical properties of packable materials are not superior to conventional hybrid composite resins, and they have shown decreased wear resistance [37]. Because packable composites do not have substantially better mechanical properties than hybrid composites, they would not be expected to perform better clinically [38,39]. In addition, because of the development of improved placement instruments and matrix systems to achieve better interproximal contacts, the need for packable or condensable materials has decreased, resulting in a decreased market share. In summary, the mechanical properties of the packable composites are not significantly better than other hybrid formulations, and there have not been sufficient long-term clinical studies to determine how these materials will perform long-term in the oral cavity. Their use as a direct dental restorative may be limited. Examples of packable composite resins in this category are Surefil (Dentsply Caulk, Milford, Deleware), Prodigy Condensable (Kerr, Orange, California), P-60 (3M, St. Paul, Minnesota), and Aelite LS Posterior (Bisco).

Compomers (polyacid modified resin composites)

Compomers are basically polyacid modified resins with filler constituents derived from composite and glass ionomer compositions. The resultant material is a low–fluoride-releasing resin composite. Compomer resins contain vinyl groups that can be polymerized by visible light activated initiators. The glass ionomer reaction within the compomer requires fluids from the oral cavity to diffuse into the composite [40]. Fluoride is able to diffuse out of the composite after the fluids swell the composite and open up the polymer networks. The fluoride release from compomers is relatively low compared with conventional glass ionomers or resin-modified glass ionomers [41]. The fluoride release and mechanical properties of compomers vary considerably between materials. Hytac (ESPE AG, Seefeld, Germany) has low fluoride release and high mechanical properties similar to resin composite. Other compomers—Compoglass (Vivadent [Ivoclar]), Dyract (Dentsply Caulk, Milford, Delaware), and F2000 (3M-Espe, St. Paul, Minnesota)—have properties more like resin-modified glass ionomers [42]. Although the manufacturer of Dyract does not recommend acid etching before the placement of the adhesive Prime & Bond NT (Dentsply Caulk), some studies have shown a low retention rate and microleakage without the acid etching step [43–45].

Conclusions from the aforementioned compomer studies make the acid etching step an absolute necessity to improve the retention rate and decrease marginal leakage. As a result, compomers must be placed exactly like traditional resin composites. Although some mechanical properties are inferior to traditional composites, recent improvements in compomer formulations such as Dyract AP (Dentsply Caulk) with a reduced filler size of 0.8 microns have improved their handling, polishability, and stain resistance. Many clinicians prefer compomers for use in Class V situations, especially if enamel is available for bonding and a limited fluoride release is desirable. Compomers are indicated for other esthetic clinical situations where they will not be subjected to significant occlusal loads [46]. These materials absorb water from the oral cavity after a period of time, so some expansion may make up for the early polymerization shrinkage [46]; however, the adhesive layer limits the uptake of the fluoride into surrounding tooth structure. The overall success of these restorations may be a result of the CTE for compomers closely matching that of tooth structure. This is important for the ability of the material to maintain marginal integrity following thermal stressing in the oral cavity.

Flowable compomers have been used clinically on a limited basis similar to flowable composites in proximal boxes for Class II restorations. One study determined that the flowable compomer Dyract Flow (Dentsply Caulk) demonstrated the least amount of overall leakage under its packable composite counterpart, compared with other flowable composite combinations [47].

Repair of composites

According to a survey of North American dental schools by the Journal of the American Dental Association, marginal defects, discoloration, and secondary caries are the most common indications for composite repair [48]. Repair of a resin-based composite restoration promotes preservation of tooth structure as well as reducing potential harmful effects on the pulp.

Composite repair may be accomplished if a patient has a localized defect. For areas not easily accessible, a preparation must be created to uncover the area of interest. In some cases a matrix band may be needed to allow adaptation of the repair resin.

Composite may be directly added if a void is detected before contouring is initiated. Because of the oxygen-inhibited surface layer, this addition is allowed, and an excellent bond between the two materials will be obtained; however, once contouring or finishing has begun, the area must be etched and adhesive placed before adding more composite to the restoration [2].

It has been reported that bonding agents and other surface treatments can be used to obtain repair strengths that are up to 80% of the cohesive strength of the material [40]. Additional factors that influence interfacial bond strength are the viscosity of the bonding resin, age of substrate resin, filler concentration and types, voids, and resin formulation [49–52]. Using different burs is likely to create differences in smearing, roughness, and matrix cracking of the existing composite. These factors also influence bond strength and micromechanical retention between the new and existing composite [53]. Flowable composites may be an attractive material for use in repair of composites, because of their low viscosity and wetting potential.

Survival probability of composites

Changes in restorative treatment patterns, the introduction of new and improved restorative materials and techniques, effective preventive programs, enhanced dental care, and growing interest in caries-free teeth have greatly influenced the longevity of dental restorations [54]; however, failure of restorations is a major problem in a practice treating primarily permanent teeth. Studies show that 60% of all operative work done is attributed to the replacement of restorations [55]. Composites have improved since their introduction, and their survival rates are improving. Clinical studies to evaluate the latest composite technologies have not been published; therefore most of the survival data are on older composite compositions.

In the 1970s, degradation or wear was considered the main reason for failure of composite restorations. Improvements in filler technology and formulation of composite materials have resulted in new reasons for replacement. Twenty years later, studies revealed secondary caries to be the new cause of failure. The main factors responsible for the change in reasons for replacement include improved clinical technique based on more adequate teaching of posterior composites at dental schools, and on gained experience through trial and error of clinicians in practice [56,57]. Advancements in composite properties and adhesive technology also contributed to these changes.

In comparison of survival probability between amalgam and composite, a time period involving 3, 4, 5, and 7 years was considered [52]. In permanent teeth, the following values were measured: 3 year, 97.2% (amalgam) to 90% (composite); 4 year, 96.6% (amalgam) to 85.6% (composite); 5 year, 95.4% (amalgam) to 78.2% (composite); and 7 year, 94.5% (amalgam) to 67.4% (composite).

In summary, longevity of composite restorations depends upon factors involving the materials, the patient, and the dentist. The request for these esthetic, tooth-colored restorations will continue to increase, and patients must be educated about the expected life of these restorations as well as their advantages and disadvantages, so they can make an informed decision on a treatment option.

Direct composite restoratives and smile design

The practice of dentistry has changed significantly in the past 2 decades. The older perceptions of dentists and previous treatment regimens have been replaced with extensive media coverage of cosmetic dentistry and the various options to improve a patient's smile. The public is more knowledgeable of cosmetic dentistry and elective esthetic treatment options. To accommodate patient's desires, dentists are incorporating smile consultation into their new patient programs. This approach focuses on the esthetic concerns of the patient, as well as showcasing cosmetic dentistry. The process includes a patient questionnaire, measurement of proportions of a patient's face, color analysis, photos, and diagnostic models [58].

The smile design approach is a comprehensive plan to fit a patients' desires. Patients have the opportunity to work with dentists to explain how they feel about their smile, teeth, gingiva, and all associated structures. Clinicians discuss numerous details, including color and size of teeth, gingival architecture, revitalizing old restorations, and other options to enhance a patient's smile [59]. Treatment options may include whitening for tooth discoloration, crown lengthening for altered passive eruption, orthognathic surgery for maxillary excess, or orthodontics to redistribute spaces between teeth before veneers [60,61]. Patients are actively involved in the treatment process by selecting options that fit their schedules, lifestyles, and personal finances.

If a patient is considering altering some aspects of her smile with composite resin or fixed prosthodontic appliances, dentists can offer tooth whitening to enhance the base color of the natural teeth, such as vital whitening or nonvital whitening for endodontically discolored teeth. The whitening (bleaching) effects on composite resin restorations may include increased wear and marginal leakage, compromising the integrity of the restoration, although these effects have not been demonstrated under short-term whitening treatment [62]. Current recommendations include replacing or refinishing composite resin restorations directly in contact with the whitening material after completion of the whitening regimen, if any question of marginal integrity exists. Composite resin restorations are more affordable than many porcelain counterparts, can be placed chairside without laboratory fees, and are easily repaired when required. Composite resin has become the material of choice for both anterior and posterior direct restorations. Manufacturers have shades specific for dentin, enamel, and tints. There are also translucent and opaque shades that can be used in a layering technique to mimic the opacity of dentin, and the translucency of enamel. These materials can also be used to create a custom shade tab directly on the tooth to allow the patient to approve of the shade before the placement of the direct restoration. Dentists often perform a mock-up composite restoration, etching the teeth so patients can see their diastema closed, or their teeth reshaped, before the actual bonding procedure. This procedure can also be performed on diagnostic stone casts to show patients the potential improvements in their smile.

For large restorations, an impression can be made to allow fabrication of an indirect composite resin restoration at a commercial laboratory. These indirect composites are polymerized extra-orally to improve the degree of conversion of the matrix resin. Indirect composites can be used to fabricate inlays and onlays for posterior teeth, veneers, and resin-bonded bridges for missing anterior teeth. The definitive restorations are bonded to the teeth with a dual cure composite resin cement. Composite resin is also used to make temporary prostheses for crowns and bridges while patients are healing from surgeries, or waiting for permanent restorations to be fabricated [63]. Composite resin has made achieving a desired esthetic result easier, more cost effective, and with wider varieties of clinical applications in dentistry.

Summary

The science and technology of composite dental restorative materials have advanced considerably over the past 10 years. Although composites have not evolved to the point of totally replacing amalgam, they have become a viable substitute for amalgam in many clinical situations. Problems still exist with polymerization contraction stress, large differences in the CTE of composites compared with tooth structure, and some technique sensitivity; however, new expanding resins, nanofiller technology, and improved bonding systems have the potential to reduce these problems. With increased patient demands for esthetic restorations, the use of direct filling composite materials will continue to grow. The one major caveat to this prediction is that clinicians must continue to use sound judgment on when, where, and how to use composite restoratives in their practice.

References

[1] Murchison DF, Roeters J, Vargas MA, et al. Direct anterior restorations. In: Summitt JB, et al, editors. Fundamentals of operative dentistry: a contemporary approach. 3rd edition. Hanover Park (IL): Quintessence Publishing Co, Inc.; 2006. p. 261–88.

[2] Roberson TM, Heymann HO, Ritter AV. Introduction to composite restorations. In: Roberson TM, Heymann HO, Swift EJ, editors. Sturdevant's art and science of operative dentistry. 4th edition. Philadelphia: Mosby Inc.; 2002. p. 471–500.

[3] Rawls HR, Upshaw JE. Restorative resins. In: Anusavice KJ, editor. Phillip's science of dental materials. 11th edition. Philladelphia: WB Saunders; 2003. p. 399–441.

[4] Bowen RJ. Synthesis of a silica-resin filling material progress report [abstract]. J Dent Res 1958;27:90.

[5] Bowen RJ. Dental filling material comprising vinyl silane treated fused silica and a binder consisting of the reaction product of bisphenol and glycidyl acrylate. US Patent 1962; 306–12.

[6] Roulet JF. Polymer constructions used in restorative dentistry. In: Degradation of dental polymers. New York: Karger; 1987. p. 3–59.

[7] Taira M, Suzaki H, Wakasa K, et al. Preparation of pure silica-glass filler for dental composites by the sol-gel process. Journal of British Ceramics Transactions 1990;89:203–7.

[8] Chen MH, Chen CR, Hsu SH, et al. Low shrinkage light curable nanocomposite for dental restorative material. Dent Mater 2006;22:138–45.

[9] Kleverlaan CJ, Feilzer AJ. Polymerization shrinkage and contraction stress of dental resin composites. Dent Mater 2006;21:1150–5.

[10] Miller MB. Reality: the information source for esthetic dentistry. Houston (TX): Reality Publishing Company; 2006.

[11] Gwinnett AJ, Kanca JA. Micromorphology of the bonded dentin interface and its relationship to bond strength. Am J Dent 1992;5:73–7.

[12] Roberson TM, Heymann HO, Ritter AV, et al. Classes I, II, and VI direct composite and other tooth-colored restorations. In: Roberson TM, Heymann HO, Swift EJ, editors. Sturdevant's art and science of operative dentistry. 4th edition. Philadelphia: Mosby Inc.; 2002. p. 471–500.

[13] Stansbury JW. Spiro orthocarbonate substituted methacrylates: new monomers for ring opening polymerization [abstract]. J Dent Res 1992;77:239.

[14] Stansbury JW. Synthesis and evaluation of new oxaspiro monomers for double ring-opening polymerization. J Dent Res 1992;71:1408–12.

[15] Eick JD, Smith RE, Pinzino CS, et al. Photopolymerization of developmental monomers for dental cationically initiated matrix resins. Dent Mater 2005;21:384–90.

[16] Anusavice KJ, Brantley WA. Physical properties of dental materials. In: Anusavice KJ, editor. Phillip's science of dental materials. 11th edition. Philadelphia: WB Saunders; 2003. p. 41–71.

[17] Thompson MN, Puckett AD, Phillips SM, et al. Heat generation from light curing units [abstract]. Presented at the Academy of Dental Materials. Southampton (Bermuda), November 11–12, 1994.

[18] Bennett B, Puckett AD, Pettey D, et al. Temperature effects on the conversion of dental composite resins. Presented at the Academy of Dental Materials. Southampton (Bermuda), November 11–12, 1994.

[19] Ferracane J. Materials in dentistry: materials and applications. 2nd edition. Baltimore (MD): Lippincott Publishing; 2001. p. 101.

[20] Chen RCS, Chan DCN, Chan KC. A quantitative study of finishing and polishing techniques for a composite. J Prosthet Dent 1988;59:291–8.

[21] Tyas MJ. Correlation between fracture properties and clinical performance of resins in Class IV cavities. Aust Dent J 1990;35:46–9.

[22] Leinfelder KF, Taylor DF, Barkmeir WW, et al. Quantitative wear measurement of posterior composite resins. Dent Mater 1986;2:198–201.

[23] Bayne S, Thompson JY, Swift EJ. A characterization of first-generation flowable composites. J Am Dent Assoc 1998;129:567–77.

[24] Xu X, Xin X, Weathersby J, et al. In vitro wear and toothbrush abrasion of flowable and posterior dental composites. J Dent Res 2002;81(special issue):A-258.

[25] Leevailoj C, Cochran MA, Matis BA, et al. Microleakage of posterior packable resin composites with and without flowable liners. Oper Dent 2001;26:302–7.

[26] Hilton TJ, Quinn R. Marginal leakage of Class II composite/flowable restorations with varied cure technique [abstract 502]. J Dent Res 2001;80:589.

[27] Jain P, Belcher M. Microleakage of Class II resin-based composite restorations with flowable composite in the proximal box. Am J Dent 2000;13:235–8.

[28] Wibowo G, Stockton L. Microleakage of Class II composite restorations. Am J Dent 2001; 14:177–85.

[29] Braga RR, Hilton TJ, Ferracane JL. Contraction stress of flowable composite materials and their efficacy as stress-relieving layers. J Am Dent Assoc 2003;134:721–8.

[30] Puetzfeldt A, Asmussen E. Composite restorations: influence of flowable and self-curing resin composite linings on microleakage in vitro. Oper Dent 2002;27(6):569–75.

[31] Ferracane JL, Berge HX, Condon JR. In vitro aging of dental composites in water—effect of degree of conversion, filler volume, and filler/matrix coupling. J Biomed Mater Res 1998; 42(3):465–72.

[32] Albers, Harry F. Tooth-colored restoratives: principles and techniques. 9th edition. Hamilton (Ontario): BC Decker; 2002. p. 120–21.

[33] Burgess JO, Walker W, Davidson JM. Posterior resin-based composite: review of the literature. Pediatr Dent 2002;24:465–79.

[34] Ferracane JL. Current trends in dental composite. Crit Rev Oral Biol Med 1995;6(4):302–18.

[35] Swift EJ. Nanocomposites. J Esthet Restor Dent 2005;17:3–4.

[36] Brackett W, Covey D. Resistance to condensation of "condensable" resin composites by a mechanical test. Oper Dent 2000;25:424–6.

[37] CRA. Condensable restorative resins. Clin Res Assoc News letter 1998;22(7):1.

[38] Leinfelder KF, Bayne SC, Swift EJ Jr. Packable composites: overview and technical considerations. J Esthet Restor Dent 1999;11(5):234–49.

[39] Cobb DS, MacGregor KM, Vargas MA, et al. The physical properties of packable and conventional posterior resin-based composites: a comparison. J Am Dent Assoc 2000;131(11): 1610–5.

[40] Kugel G. Direct and indirect adhesive restorative materials: a review. Am J Dent 2000; 13(special issue):350–400.

[41] Burgess JO, Norling BK, Rawls HR, et al. Directly placed esthetic restorative materials—the continuum. Compend Contin Educ Dent 1996;17:731–48.

[42] Iazetti G, Burgess JO, Gardiner D. Selected mechanical properties of fluoride releasing materials. Oper Dent 2001;26:21–6.

[43] Jedynakiewicz N, Martin N. A three year evaluation of a compomer restoration [abstract]. J Dent Res 1997;76:162.

[44] Triana R, Prado C, Garro J, et al. Dentin bond strength of fluoride-releasing materials. Am J Dent 1994;7(5):252–4.

[45] Kugel G, Perry RD, Hoang E, et al. Dyract compomer: comparison of total etch vs. no etch technique. Gen Dent 1998;46(6):604–6.

[46] Mount GJ. Description of glass-ionomers. In: An atlas of glass-ionomer cements: a clinician's guide. 3rd edition. London: Martin Dunitz Ltd; 2002. p. 1–42.

[47] Neme AL, Maxson BB, Pink FE, et al. Microleakage of Class II packable resin composites lined with flowables: an in vitro study study. Oper Dent 2002;27(6):600–5.

[48] Gordan VV, Mjor IA, Blum IR, et al. Teaching students the repair of resin-based composite restorations: a survey of North American dental schools. J Am Dent Assoc 2003;134:317–23.

[49] Gregory WA, Pounder B, Bakus E. Bond strengths of chemically dissimilar repaired composite resins. J Prosthet Dent 1990;64:664–8.

[50] Powers JM, Pratten DH, Collard SM, et al. Spreading of oligomers on polymers. Dent Mater 1991;7:88–91.

[51] Puckett AD, Holder R, O'Hara JW. Strength of posterior composite repairs using different composite/bonding agent combinations. Oper Dent 1991;16:136–40.

[52] Pounder B, Gregory WA, Powers JM. Bond strengths of repaired composite resins. Oper Dent 1987;12:127–31.

[53] DeSchepper EJ, Tate WH, Powers JM. Bond strength of resin cements to microfilled composites. J Dent 1993;6:235–8.

[54] Kejici I, Lutz F. Marginal adaptation of Class V restorations using different restorative techniques. J Dent 1991;19:24–32.

[55] Mjor IA. Amalgam and composite resin resin restorations: longevity and reasons for replacement. In: Anusavice K, editor. Quality of evaluation of dental restorations. Chicago: Quintessence Publishing Corp, Inc.; 1989. p. 61–80.

[56] Mjor IA, Wilson NHF. The teaching of Class I and Class II direct composite restorations in North American dental schools. J Am Dent Assoc 1998;129:1415–21.

[57] Wilson NHF, Mjor IA. The teaching of Class I and Class II direct composite restorations in European dental schools. J Dent 2000;26:15–21.

[58] Aschein KW, King MP. Eshtetics and oral photography. In: Ascheim KW, Dale BG, editors. Esthetic dentistry: a clinical approach to techniques and materials. St. Louis (MO): Mosby Inc.; 2001. p. 269–87.

[59] Chadwick BL, Dummer PMH, Dunstan F, et al. The longevity of dental restorations: a systematic review. National Health Service Centre for Reviews and Dissemination. University of York (UK); 2001.

[60] Chiche GJ, Pinault A. Esthetics of anterior fixed prosthodontics. Chicago: Quintessence Publishing Co, Inc.; 1994.

[61] Goldstein RE. Change your smile. 3rd edition. Chicago: Quintessence Publishing Co, Inc.; 1997.

[62] Heyman H. Additional conservative esthetic procedures. In: Roberson TM, Heymann HO, Swift EJ, editors. Sturdevant's art and science of operative dentistry. 4th edition. Philadelphia: Mosby Inc.; 2002. p. 608–12.

[63] Chiche GJ, Aoshima H. Smile design: a guide for clinician, ceramist, and patient. Chicago: Quintessence Publishing Co, Inc.; 2004.

ELSEVIER
SAUNDERS

Dent Clin N Am 51 (2007) 677–694

THE DENTAL
CLINICS
OF NORTH AMERICA

Adhesion to Tooth Structure Mediated by Contemporary Bonding Systems

Ivan Stangel, DMD[a,b,*], Thomas H. Ellis, PhD[c],
Edward Sacher, PhD[d]

[a]*BioMat Sciences, 5612 Glenwood Road, Bethesda, MD 20817, USA*
[b]*McGill University, Faculty of Dentistry, 3640 University Street, Montréal,
Québec, Canada H3A 2B2*
[c]*Synchrotron Light Source, University of Saskatchewan,
101 Perimeter Road, Saskatoon, Saskatchewan, S7N 0X4, Canada*
[d]*Department of Engineering Physics, École Polytechnique, C.P. 6079,
Succursale Centre-Ville, Montréal, Québec H3C 3A7, Canada*

The achievement of high-strength, durable bonds between tooth structure and restorative materials has been a long-term goal of the dental profession. The formation of such bonds would lead to a true surgical model of operative treatment of teeth and the universal application of minimally invasive dentistry. In principle, operative intervention would only require the removal of the diseased or undermined parts of teeth. Subsequent reconstruction for the long-term would be based on the use of a restorative material retained only by an adhesive system, whether in load or non–load-bearing environments. This approach provides the advantages of (1) work simplification, (2) reduced treatment time, (3) reduced biological cost, (4) an ability to retain restorative materials without any form of retention, including pins and posts, and (5) an improvement in the quality of the interface between materials and tooth walls.

Although it took more than 20 years to become widely accepted, Buonocore established the basis for modern restorative dentistry in 1955, when he described a technique for bonding acrylic materials to enamel using phosphoric acid [1]. More than two decades later, the strength of adhesive joints formed by bonding resins to etched enamel resulted in the widespread use of acid-etching techniques rather than pins for the retention of class IV composite restorations [2,3]. Thus began the era of adhesive dentistry.

Parts of this work were supported by the Natural Sciences and Engineering Research Council of Canada.
* Corresponding author. BioMat Sciences, 5612 Glenwood Road, Bethesda, MD 20817.
E-mail address: stangel@biomatsciences.com (I. Stangel).

After nearly three decades of experience, adhesive techniques are routinely incorporated into clinical practice. Acid treatment of enamel or dentin, whether an a priori or concomitant bonding step, has been integrated into methods to retain materials and significantly reduce microleakage at material-tooth interfaces [4]. In addition to tooth reconstruction, a multiplicity of adhesive clinical procedures—ranging from fissure sealants to laminate veneering to resin bonded bridges—has been spawned. Little did Buonocore appreciate the impact of his discovery on the quality of care more than 50 years later.

Given the enormity of the field of adhesion and the number of commercial products available, the discipline of modern adhesive dentistry can be daunting with respect to materials and techniques. This article organizes contemporary bonding practice and materials around an understanding of the fundamentals of adhesion to tooth structure. In providing this context, adhesive development, bonding systems, and their appropriate use are better understood. The end result is the better practice of adhesive dentistry.

Adhesion basics

In descriptive terminology, adhesion is the bonding or the attachment of dissimilar materials. When applied to surfaces, adhesives join materials together to resist separation and transmit loads across the bonds. The materials being joined are commonly referred to as substrates or adherends.

Adhesion is not an inherent property of an adhesive. Rather, it is the response of an assembly to deformation loads. In the dental literature, this is often referred to as "bond strength." When stress is applied to the assembly, energy is absorbed. The adhesive transfers and distributes the stress to the components of the joint. The strain response to the stress is a manifestation of the properties of all the materials that comprise the assembly.

Failure of assemblies (eg, composite-tooth joints) occurs as a result of flaws, which propagate under stress as cracks and can originate in any component of the assembly. The ability of an assembly to resist crack growth is a function of its toughness. Although "bond strength" is commonly used in the dental literature, a load being applied is often attenuated by the adherends before load transfer to the bond. For example, the modulus, or stiffness of those adherends, rather than the strength of the adhesive can vary the result of a "bond strength" test. For conventional tests of dental bonding systems, such as the commonly used shear test, cracks often initiate in one of the adherends. In these cases, although results are often referred to as "bond strength," the intrinsic strength of the bond layer is not quantified. Rather, the strength of the adhesive joint is measured. A better term for describing these types of tests is "adhesive joint strength."

The microtensile bond test was developed to overcome this problem by designing samples to concentrate stress to the bond layer of an assembly.

Here, test failure always occurs at the adhesive level. Information about the strength inherent to bonding materials rather than the adherends is generated. The microtensile test is more cumbersome and more difficult to undertake than some of the conventional tests; however, the insights gained are thought to outweigh these issues [5]. Because of increased difficulty in sample preparation and testing, conventional tests, such as shear bond strength, are still used and reported in the literature [6,7].

Microtensile tests use multiple samples from a single tooth-composite assembly. For example, if eight specimens are obtained from a single assembly, this data set is treated as a sample of size eight by many researchers. This approach may not be appropriate with respect to managing experimental variation and analysis, however. Consequently, conclusions from bond strength studies in which adequate sample size has not been used may not be supported by the data. Appropriate sample size management and increasing the number of experimental units (tooth-composite assemblies) provide better reliability of conclusions drawn from the vast literature on adhesives [8].

Adhesion promotion

The survival rate of no-preparation bonded cervical composite restorations in at least some short-term clinical trials has been shown to range from 45% to 100% [9]. That restoration retention occurs at all by only applying solutions to tooth surfaces—and that it varies significantly—speaks to phenomena that occur at the interface between materials and tooth structure. These phenomena are largely based on surface reactions of those solutions with tooth structure. The elucidation of these surface reactions provides a good starting point for appreciating contemporary commercial bonding systems.

Whether bonding composites to tooth structure or paint to steel, two primary variables are to be considered in the formation of bonds between dissimilar materials. The first of these variables is the substrate being bonded to, and the second involves the nature of materials that interfacially interact with those surfaces. Their interactions and the properties of the materials used are the major determinants for the long-term success of the adhesive joints formed. In all cases, adhesion promotion follows a prescribed generic methodology, which involves (1) substrate preparation, (2) the application of functional molecules (primers) to the surface, and (3) the placement of application-specific overlayers that react with the primer.

Each step in the methodology has a specific function. Substrate optimization involves the dissolution of barrier layers that inhibit primer interaction with the intended bulk material (ie, the material to which bonds are to be formed). In some cases, these layers are measured in angstroms, as in the case of an oxide layer or multilayer. (As a point of reference, a sheet of paper is approximately 1 million Å thick.) In heterogeneous materials (eg, enamel and dentin), surface preparation also can involve the selective removal of substrate components to enable more efficient surface reactions, alter surface conformation, or change the surface energy [10].

Optimization of tooth surfaces involves the use of acids for the removal of smear debris (the barrier layer on tooth surfaces) and the dissolution of apatite crystals from enamel and dentin (the selective removal of substrate components) to develop microporous surfaces. Acid treatment also modifies the surface energy, which can be easily observed by placing a drop of water on either enamel or dentin before and after acid treatment. In the "before" case, the drop of water is observed to "bead up" and have a relatively large contact angle. After acid treatment, the water spreads on the surface and has a contact angle that is effectively as low as zero.

In general, primers are bi- or multifunctional molecules with chemical group terminations that react with the adherends. In dental applications, primer molecules have an "adhesive" group at one end to react with enamel or dentin and a polymerizable group at the other end to cross-link with resin overlayers, typically known as "bonding" or "adhesive" resins. Variations of phosphorous-containing functionalities have been the most common feature of adhesive groups, although other functionalities, such as carboxylic acids, have been shown to be useful. The adhesive and polymerizable ends of the primer are separated by a "spacer," which determines many of the properties of the primer, including solubility and wetting [11,12].

The function of a primer when bonding to enamel is to wet the surface (one of the requirements for promoting strong adhesion) and penetrate microporosities. In dentin, in addition to wetting, primers diffuse through the surface of the demineralized region and entangle collagen fibers on polymerization. Primers also can react with functional groups inherent to collagen or with apatite inherent to enamel or at the front between unaltered and demineralized dentin.

Resin overlayers copolymerize with primers and with subsequently placed composite resins. They have extensive cross-linking capabilities and add considerable strength to the adhesive joint. They are typically composed of comonomers, each of which contributes specific beneficial properties to the formation of the adhesive joint. Resin overlayers also can bond mechanically to other materials, such as amalgam, when using amalgam-bonding techniques.

Nomenclature

Historically, bonding systems have been composed of components that were applied sequentially and followed the generic adhesion promotion steps previously outlined. To simplify bonding procedures and reduce the reporting of postoperative sensitivity (the latter being thought to result from incomplete permeation of primers in demineralized dentin), steps were combined. Adhesive systems based on various permutations of the application steps were developed, including adhesives that combined the generic steps one and two, or two and three, or even steps one, two, and three into a single solution.

In contemporary nomenclature, bonding systems are classified by whether an acidic solution is applied and rinsed or left in situ. These are respectively referred to as "etch-and-rinse" or "no-rinse" systems. The former is composed of either three- or two-step systems, in which the initial step always involves a neat acid application. The etch-and-rinse two-step system is sometimes referred to as a one-bottle system, despite the need for two steps. The one-bottle system is composed of a solution that contains primer and adhesive resin components.

No-rinse systems, generically referred to as self-etch bonding materials, can either involve two- or one-step applications. The former application demineralizes and primes tooth surfaces simultaneously. The adhesive layer is applied as a second step. One-step bonding materials demineralize, prime, and bond in a single application. With the exception of glass ionomer cements, whose carboxyl functionality complexes with calcium in apatite [13], all adhesive systems used by dental professionals follow the generic bonding methodology described. The systems differ from each other with respect to application steps and specific composition used for achieving each of the adhesion promotion objectives. These differences account for their differences in clinical performance.

Substrate structure

Although well characterized elsewhere, a brief discussion of tooth substrates is useful with respect to a more detailed discussion of surface reactions of bonding systems.

Enamel

Compositionally, enamel contains 96% inorganic matter by weight, the balance being water and organic material [14]. The latter consists of proteins in the form of amelogenins and enamelins. The inorganic matter consists of hydroxyapatite, a crystalline form of calcium phosphate, although some carbonate is present. Collectively, they are referred to as biological apatite [15]. Structurally, enamel is composed of a higher order structure that consists of "rods," which are organized in a repetitive pattern referred to as a "head-and-tail" arrangement. Crystal organization within the rod is complex, with crystal orientation varying based on location [16].

Dentin

Dentin is considerably more complex and consists of solid and porous phases. The porous phase consists of numerous fluid-filled tubules emanating from the pulp. They traverse the dentin to the dentino-enamel junction, making dentin a highly permeable tissue. Each dentinal tubule is surrounded by a collar of hypermineralized, peritubular dentin [17]. The organic matrix of peritubular dentin is delicate and is lost along the mineral phase after decalcification. The structure surrounding the peritubular dentin is intertubular dentin, which is approximately 9% less mineralized than peritubular dentin.

Intertubular dentin constitutes the bulk of the solid phase of dentin. The intertubular dentin is a biphasic biologic composite that contains mineral and organic components. As in enamel, the mineral phase consists of crystals of biologic apatite, although dentinal hydroxyapatite is plate-shaped and much smaller than the hydroxyapatite crystal in enamel [15]. The organic phase of dentin primarily consists of type I collagen, which acts as a scaffold for mineralization, and minor amounts of noncollagenous proteins, which are implicated in mineralization [18]. Collagen is generally acid insoluble [19], whereas noncollagenous proteins are soluble in the acids used for tooth demineralization (Ivan Stangel, DMD, unpublished data, 1996). The dentin matrix remains relatively intact after decalcification, whereas noncollagenous proteins are removed from their surfaces.

Surface reactions: acid effects

Adhesion promotion to mineralized tissue is based on the reaction of biologic apatite with acids. For water-soluble acids, the nature of the reaction and the degree of demineralization are complex and are based on pH and counterion. In dentin, the reaction kinetics are diffusion controlled [15]. Although proton concentration can correlate directly to the degree of demineralization, the solubility of calcium salts (reaction products) at the demineralization front affects the degree of demineralization [15,17]. For example, for a given pH, maleic acid produces a deeper demineralized region in dentin than does citric acid, partly because of the formation of insoluble salts at the demineralization front [20]. For water-soluble salts, an increase in pH increases the degree of demineralization according to the general reaction in the following equation [21]:

$$Ca_{10}(PO)_6 + H^+ \rightarrow Ca^{2+} + \text{phosphate species} + H_2O$$

This reaction has implications for the integrity of adhesion to enamel for certain acidic primers with respect to proton concentration and the ability to sufficiently demineralize tooth surfaces. Milder self-etch adhesives have a lower proton concentration, which affects the quality of etch on enamel and dentin.

In essence, acid reaction with either enamel or dentin dissolves apatite crystals and creates a microporous surface morphology. In the case of enamel, the rate of dissolution depends on crystal orientation-inter-rod rather than rod peripheries are preferentially removed to produce the microporous surface. The chemical composition of this surface, when using water soluble acids, remains comparable to native enamel.

In the case of dentin, acid treatment removes the smear layer, exposes collagen, increases dentin permeability, and chemically modifies the surface [10,15]. A microporous surface is also formed. However, here it is predominantly composed of a complex network of collagen fibrils largely absent of mineral crystals and containing significant amounts of water that has displaced apatite crystals. In addition to demineralizing effects, the application of phosphoric acid to dentin surfaces removes acid-soluble phosphoproteins that are implicated in mineralization of collagen surfaces [22].

Thus, the basis for most adhesion in modern dentistry involves the reaction of biological apatites with protons and the subsequent secondary reactions that occur with priming agents. The manner of applications of the agents and the nature of the materials designed to interact with the acid-treated surfaces are what distinguish the modern bonding systems.

Mechanisms of adhesion

The mechanisms of adhesion to the inorganic and organic components of teeth have relied primarily on the evaluation of morphologic relationships of materials with tooth substrates. As of this writing, a literature search on Pub Med using the key words [morphology dental bonding] returned 3300 "hits." Although they make major contributions to understanding phenomena relating to adhesion, theories based only on microscopic examination of resin-tooth interfaces fail to consider potential chemical adhesion, inasmuch as the elucidation of molecular interactions cannot be determined by microscopy. Surface-sensitive techniques using various spectroscopies have been used to elucidate reactions between tooth structure and materials used for adhesive bonding. These techniques are described subsequently.

Enamel

Bonding to enamel can occur through either the well-known micromechanical retention of polymers on etched surfaces or chemical bonding to apatite. For the former approach, the gold standard for demineralizing enamel is highly concentrated (generally, pH < 1.0) phosphoric acid having a concentration on the order of 35 weight percent. When coated with primers and subsequently placed resin overlayers, the ensuing micromechanical bond to phosphoric-acid etched enamel is substantial. The in vitro strength of adhesive joints formed by composite resins bonded to etched enamel has been reported to be on the order of 27 MPa [23].

Self-etching primers use an acidic primer to demineralize enamel surfaces. Primers can be made acidic by grafting on carboxylic acid or a phosphate ester. The pH of self-etching primers ranges from aggressive to mild (approximately 0.4–2.5). As would be expected, the etch patterns of the milder systems on uncut enamel are not as profound as those with a more aggressive etch [24]. The latter system produces etch patterns consistent with total-etch systems.

Whether an aggressive or mild etch pattern, the microtensile bond strength of no-rinse, self-etching systems on uncut enamel tends to be less than that of a conventional etch-and-rinse system [25]. On ground enamel, the bond strength for some self-etching systems improves but does not approach the strength and reliability of etch-and-rinse systems [26]. Consistently, the highest bond strengths to enamel are obtained with an a priori etch and remain the standard against which all other systems are compared.

The use of a prior acid application step (to be rinsed off) increases bond strength to enamel for at least some no-rinse, self-etching adhesives and is recommended when restorations primarily rely on bonds to enamel formed to enamel [27,28]. The application of phosphoric acid to dentin diminishes the bonding efficacy of self-etching adhesives to dentin, however [29]. Effective bonding to noncarious sclerotic dentin in the cervical region of teeth also may require enhanced demineralization capability [30]. The use of mild self-etching adhesives may preclude predictable bonding for no-preparation restorations.

In addition to micromechanical bonding, bonding to enamel apatite can occur through complexation with the calcium ion or reaction with the phosphate or the hydroxyl groups [31]. Reactions along these lines occur with the treatment of enamel by polyalkenoic acids [32]. The complexation of carboxyl groups derived from polyalkenoic acid with calcium is ionic in nature and may not be substantial for clinical use. Improvement in the glass ionomer bond to enamel can be made by pretreating surfaces with polyalkenoic acid [33]. The effect of the acid, as with other acids, is to remove smear layer and partially demineralize the enamel surface. In addition to ionic bond formation to apatite, a micromechanical component to the bond is obtained [34].

Dentin

The hybridization theory originally advanced by Nakabayashi [35] is the most commonly accepted basis for adhesion to dentin. Acid demineralization of superficial dentin exposes a collagen fibril network having inter- and intrafibrillar microporosities. Low-viscosity monomers placed on this surface diffuse into the demineralized region to form a resin-dentin interdiffusion zone. On polymerization, entanglement of the fibrils by the resin occurs to create a hybrid layer of resin-reinforced dentin. Formation of this hybrid layer is thought to be the primary bonding mechanism for many adhesive systems [36,37]. That this is a commonly accepted mechanism may relate to the previously mentioned preponderance of studies that rely on microscopy and the morphologic evaluation of adhesive joints.

Mechanisms are more complex, however, and may involve primer solubility issues and chemical reactions with collagen, with residual apatite in dentin demineralized with mild acids, or with unaltered dentin at its interface with demineralized collagen. A secondary (possibly even a primary) bonding mechanism also may occur at the interface between demineralized and unaltered dentin. Examination of this interface demonstrates a relatively irregular surface that may inherently produce micromechanical bonds comparable to those formed to etched enamel.

The latter phenomenon can be observed in studies in which deproteination of collagen-rich demineralized dentin produces bonds that are substantial [38–40]. This occurrence indicates that at least for some adhesive systems, the presence of a conventional hybrid layer is not necessarily a requirement for producing high bond strength. It further suggests that other mechanisms of bond formation to dentin are in effect [41]. The basis for this observation needs further study.

The development of dental priming molecules has concentrated on the synthesis of phosphate derivatives of bifunctional mono- or dimethacrylate monomers. The adhesion mechanism of these structures may be based on ionic bonding of the phosphate group with one of the components of dentin. That the phosphate group may play a significant role in adhesion has been shown in a study that evaluated surface state effects on phosphate-mediated bonds to dentin [12]. In that study, dipentaerythritol pentaacrylate monophosphate (DPP) and its analog, dipentaerythritol monohydroxy-pentaacrylate (DPO), having a hydroxyl rather than a phosphate termination, were respectively bonded to (1) smeared dentin, (2) polished dentin (dentin in which the smear layer had been mechanically removed), (3) demineralized dentin, and (4) demineralized/deproteinated dentin. The adhesive joint strength for DPP was significantly greater than that of DPO at each level. The shear strength (in MPa) of the adhesive joint for DPP ranged from 22.7 to 33.1, whereas the MPa range for DPO was 0.5 to 11.1 MPa. That DPO had some low level of bond formation to polished dentin suggests that the terminal OH group has some capability of bonding to hydroxyapatite. The strength to demineralized and deproteinated dentin suggests a contribution of micromechanical bond formation.

In addition to hybridization, chemical bonding to mineral and protein components of dentin has been described [31,42–45]. Organic compounds that can bond to ions in mineral apatite found in dentin include (1) phosphate-based adhesives, (2) amino acid- or amino alcohol-based adhesives, and (3) adhesives based on dicarboxylates [46]. Compounds that contain hydroxyl, carboxyl, amino, and amido groups can potentially react with bonding sites inherent to collagen [45–47].

Type I collagen comprises approximately 90% of the organic phase of dentin. Collagen is an ordered structure whose basic unit, the collagen molecule, is composed of a triple helix, with each of its strands being composed of approximately 20 amino acids, in which every third amino acid is glycine. Potential reactive sites in collagen primarily consist of carboxylate and hydroxyl groups. The latter can be found in sufficient concentration in hydroxyproline, threonine, and serine. The former groups are found in aspartate and glutamate. Reactions to either or both of these groups could form the basis of chemical bonding to the organic phase of dentin.

Using subtractive spectroscopic techniques and surface-sensitive photoacoustic Fourier transform infrared spectroscopy and Fourier transform-Raman spectroscopies, surface reactions between hydroxyethyl methacrylate, a common component of contemporary adhesive systems, and collagen have been elaborated [31,44,45]. These reactions have been shown to involve transesterification, secondary amide formation, or possibly hydrogen bonding. It should be noted that several mechanisms of adhesion can operate simultaneously. Hybridization and chemical bond formation can work synergistically in forming bonds to dentin.

Enamel-dentinal adhesives

All contemporary adhesive systems bond to enamel or dentin through the mechanisms described. At some level, they conform to the generic steps for adhesion promotion, whether the solutions used are sequentially or concomitantly applied. What distinguishes the different classes of adhesive are the modes of application of the solutions and, within classes, the components and chemistries inherent to a particular material.

It is worth noting that one of the classification systems found in the literature is based on generational sequencing [50]. There is a belief, by at least some practitioners, that bonding systems of a more recent generation constitute advances over prior ones. However, the more recent generations are based on a reduction of the number of application steps, which is generally believed to reduce adhesive performance. It is the belief of these authors that advances in adhesion should not be classified on the basis of the number of bottles opened but rather on advances in interfacial chemistry that ultimately lead to improved performance and quality of care. It is from these advances that the goal of routine practice of minimally invasive dentistry will be achieved.

Etch-and-rinse adhesives

Three-step systems

Conventional enamel-dentin primers consist of polymerizable monomers in an organic solvent [48]. Molecular backbones have hydrophilic group terminations with an affinity to the dentin surface and hydrophobic functionalities capable of copolymerizing with resin overlayers. Additional hydrophilic comonomers are added to the solvent, given the high water content of demineralized dentin surfaces [49]. Other components include photoinitiators, stabilizers, and fillers. The primer functions to "wet" collagen fibril surfaces to the full depth of demineralization and displace water at sites at which demineralization has occurred. It also functions to react with tooth substrates and mechanically entangle collagen on polymerization.

The solvent phase for primers in three-step systems is typically organic in nature and is usually acetone or ethanol. The advantage of acetone is that it has a high vapor pressure and displaces water [50]. Solvents that effectively displace water maximize monomer diffusion into demineralized dentin, which is particularly important for demineralized dentin inasmuch as the inter- and intrafibrillar spaces of collagen formerly occupied by apatite crystals are replaced by water [51].

Acetone's high vapor pressure is an advantage and a disadvantage. As an advantage, residual solvent on bonding surfaces (which can inhibit polymerization) is readily removed. The disadvantage of high vapor pressure is that it can adversely affect bonding efficacy by changing monomer concentration during usage and storage [52]. In one study that compared acetone, ethanol, and water as solvents in one-bottle systems [53], acetone-based, one-bottle adhesives demonstrated a mass loss of 30% to 45% over a 7-day period compared with ethanol-based adhesives, which had a mass loss of 15% to 38% over the same period. This loss for acetone and ethanol seems to be rather high and is not consistent with mass loss for other acetone-based systems, which have been measured over a 45-day storage period at ambient temperature in a polypropylene container as being on the order of 1% (Ivan Stangel, DMD, unpublished data, 2006).

Ethanol and water are polar solvents and have the potential of expanding a collagen matrix that has collapsed because of drying [54]. Because the native conformation of hydrated collagen is maintained by hydrogen bonding, it is clear that the loss of water would cause collagen collapse [55]. Up to a point, the introduction of polar solvents to re-expand collagen makes sense, because their hydrogen bonding potential is high [56]. The use of adhesives that contain solvents with hydrogen-bonding potential would be useful where dentin surfaces have been allowed to dehydrate excessively.

The adhesive-resin component of a bonding system is generally composed of cross-linking methacrylates, which contribute to the strength and integrity of the bonded layer and enhance the rate of polymerization [11]. The polymer network formed is the building block between primers and filled resins, with copolymerization occurring to each of these layers. In comparison to the commonly used hydrophilic hydroxyethyl methacrylate, cross-linking methacrylates are hydrophobic and have lower water sorption. Water sorption decreases as the polymer network density increases.

The most common cross-linking methacrylates are 2,2-bis[4-(3-methacryloyloxy-2-hydroxypropoxy)phenyl]propane (bis-GMA), triethyleneglycol dimethacrylate (TEGDMA), and urethane dimethacrylate. The degree of conversion of adhesive resins is based on the specific composition of the resin, the concentration of its components, and the method used for determining degree of conversion [57]. The degree of conversion range of bis-GMA/TEGDMA systems is on the order of 50% to 70%.

Two-step systems

Two-step etch-and-rinse systems combine the primer and adhesive resin components into a single solution. Bonds formed to enamel with these systems are comparable to those formed by three-step systems, because their ability to wet and impregnate etched dentin is efficient [58]. Bonds formed to dentin are less effective, however, because incomplete diffusion of the adhesive occurs under wet bonding conditions and leaves a porous collagen network in place [59,60]. Phase separation also occurs in the interphase region between the hydrophilic primers and hydrophobic resins, which results in inhomogeneity of the adhesive-dentin interface. The degree of inhomogeneity is system dependent, with acetone-based, one-bottle systems having greater penetration than ethanol-based systems. In either case, incomplete encapsulation of collagen fibers in the demineralized region of dentin can lead to nanoleakage and subsequent bond degradation [61].

No-rinse adhesives

No-rinse adhesives were developed to overcome incomplete sealing of dentin, which was believed to be caused by technique-sensitive components of etch-and-rinse systems. The incomplete sealing was thought to be a factor in often reported postoperative sensitivity.

An approach to bonding that eliminated the acid demineralization step (to overcome the incomplete permeation of demineralized dentin with etch-and-rinse, one-bottle systems) and provide for work simplification would have advantages over the etch-and-rinse systems. Thus, the basis for self-etching adhesives was conceived. They conform to the generic steps of adhesion by demineralizing and priming in a single step, with the interfacial resin layer being placed separately, or by simultaneously demineralizing, priming, and forming interfacial layers.

Two-step/one-step systems

Two-step self-etch adhesives use polymerizable acidic monomers to simultaneously demineralize and prime tooth surfaces. The application of a hydrophilic primer is followed by a hydrophobic bond material that conforms, more or less, to the adhesive resin description provided for three-step and etch-and-rinse systems.

The most recent developments involve the promotion of adhesive systems as one-step systems. Manufacturers have combined acidic primers into a single solution that etches, primes, and bonds in one application. Acidic monomers in no-rinse systems contain a polymerizable group to copolymerize with other monomers and subsequently placed bonding resins. They also have a functional acidic group, such as a carboxylic or phosphoric acid group, to demineralize tooth surfaces and potentially chelate with intact minerals in those surfaces.

Self-etching primers use water as the primary solvent to ionize the primer. Ionization is the process that produces protons in solution for the demineralization reaction (see previous equation). As such, in principle, sensitivity to water inherent to dentin is not an issue. Because water is already present in dentin (approximately 10% by weight), however, the application of water-based, self-etching adhesives onto tooth surfaces may result in a dilution of priming components within the collagen network when mixing with water in dentin. Water also inhibits polymerization of adhesive monomers. Both phenomena reduce the integrity of the adhesive joint formed by self-etching primers, and this can be observed microscopically [62]. That this is the case is shown by in vitro strength tests that generally demonstrate lower strength for water-based adhesives compared with acetone-based adhesives [51,63].

To be functional, self-etching primers need to dissolve smear layers and aprismatic enamel to form hybrid layers with enamel and dentin. The monomers must be relatively acidic, with current two-step self-etching primers having a pH range of 1.0 to 2.5. One-step systems have a pH less than 1.0. Under these acidic conditions, esters such as hydroxyethyl methacrylate, TEGDMA, and urethane dimethacrylate are hydrolytically unstable and undergo up to 90% degradation when stored [26,64]. Such instability may lead to degradation of in vivo bonding performance.

Hydrolytic instability in solution can be reduced by reducing the acidity of the primer to a pH more than 2. This pH is considered to be relatively mild, however, and adhesives at this acidity level may not adequately etch enamel or form sufficiently deep hybrid layers in dentin. On enamel, aggressive (pH < 1.0) self-etching primers produce etch patterns that are consistent with surfaces treated with phosphoric acid [65]. The depth of demineralization for dentin also can be comparable to etch-and-rinse systems.

Regardless of the pH and etch patterns of self-etching primers, an etch-and-rinse approach to bonding to enamel generally produces significantly greater in vitro adhesive joint strength compared with self-etching primers [26]. For dentin, conventional three-step total-etch adhesives generally produce significantly higher adhesive joint strengths than either one- or two-step adhesives [66].

Adhesive evaluation

A brief discussion of the methods of evaluating bonds formed to tooth substrates is warranted. Although in vivo trials are clearly the gold standard for evaluating the performance of adhesive systems, the high cost of trials, the wide range of variables involved, and the long time periods required for data collection have led to extensive use of in vitro tests for the evaluation of adhesive materials [67]. Clinical trials also have limited value with respect to the fact that most evaluations of adhesives rely on the no-preparation class V cervical lesion. Although it can be argued that there is a reasonable amount of tensile loading in this environment because of coronal strain, cervical restorations are generally considered to be non–load-bearing. Thus, the true utility of adhesives for the universal practice of minimally invasive dentistry—whether for load- or non–load-bearing restorations—is difficult to assess in a systematic way.

Nonetheless, an excellent review of the clinical performance of dental adhesives was published recently [68]. The review used published literature from university-based clinical trials primarily involving noncarious cervical lesions. Eighty-five peer-reviewed publications and non–peer-reviewed abstracts were used for the analysis. The studies collectively evaluated three-step etch-and-rinse, two-step etch-and-rinse, two-step self-etching, and one-step self-etching adhesives and glass ionomers with and without conditioning.

There was a high degree of variability within each of the groups, whose detailed discussion is beyond the scope of this article. Briefly, however, three-step etch-and-rinse adhesives performed better than the two-step etch-and-rinse adhesives. The basis for this may relate to phase separation of one-bottle systems and incomplete infiltration of the demineralized layer [69]. Two-step self-etch adhesives showed a clinically reliable performance in non–load-bearing restorations that approached that of the three-step etch-and-rinse systems. Their annual failure rate showed a larger variation than did the latter, however. Several self-etch systems required selective enamel etching; thus, they were not true no-rinse systems. "An inefficient clinical performance" was observed for the one-step adhesives. They had the largest variability in annual clinical failures, recording from 0 to 48% restoration loss.

It should be noted that resin-modified glass ionomer performance was comparable to three-step etch-and-rinse systems. Conventional glass ionomers, however, had a loss rate that was somewhat greater than the resin-modified form.

From this analysis, several conclusions can be made. First, there is an absence of systematic data on the performance of adhesive systems in true load-bearing environments, which limits the ability to recommend with confidence the routine application of minimally invasive adhesive restorative dentistry. Anecdotal evidence may support this extended use and certainly merits the initiation of clinical trials to test the hypothesis that modern adhesive materials used under minimally invasive conditions retain restorations in load-bearing environments.

Second, there is a tendency in the literature to classify adhesives by their "generational" iteration. Many believe that this nomenclature suggests that each successive generation is an improvement over prior ones, which is not the case, as clearly shown by the analysis of clinical performance cited earlier. The latest versions of adhesives (the one-bottle self-etch systems) not only demonstrate relatively lower in vitro bond strength to enamel but also tend to have the highest rates of failure in clinical trials.

Finally, one of the bases for the development of self-etching adhesives was the anecdotal reporting of postoperative sensitivity associated with etch-and-rinse systems. If it does exist, however, the basis for postoperative sensitivity is complex and may originate from several sources, including exacerbation of pre-existing pulpal pathology, bacterial presence at the interface, polymerization shrinkage of composite resins, and alteration of fluid flow of tubules [70,71]. Because of the complexity of postoperative sensitivity, the isolation to an adhesive bonding methodology is difficult to assess without undertaking systematic clinical trials. When assessed in controlled clinical studies, no differences in postoperative sensitivity were found between self-etching and etch-and-rinse adhesives [72–74].

Utility of modern adhesive systems

In returning to the fundamental principles of adhesion, the contribution of micromechanical bonding to the formation of an adhesion cannot be underestimated. Nonetheless, it is these authors' opinion that advances in adhesion, where reliability and durability of bonds are the ultimate goal, should be based on the improved chemistry of the interface and the ability to react adhesives with tooth substrates. Such reactions can only occur when barrier layers are removed and the substrate itself is exposed. This is difficult to accomplish with no-rinse systems because calcium salts, amorphous calcium phosphate, and dissolved proteins remain as part of the monomer mixture at bonding sites.

Bonding systems applied to surfaces where such barriers are not removed likely inhibit the ability to form bonds directly with substrates. Although self-etching systems have shown excellent results for certain types of restorations, their use for universal application in minimally invasive dentistry under all clinical loading conditions is limited. New strategies must be developed that are biomimetic in nature and produce long-term, stable bonding.

References

[1] Buonocore MG. A simple method of increasing the adhesion of acrylic filling materials to enamel surfaces. J Dent Res 1955;34(6):849–53.
[2] Gilpatrick RQ, Ross JA, Simonsen RJ. Resin-to-enamel bond strength with various etching times. Quintessence Int 1991;22(1):47–9.
[3] Gwinnett AJ, Kanca J. Micromorphology of the bonded dentin interface and its relationship to bond strength. Am J Dent 1992;5(2):73–7.
[4] Shaffer SE, Barkmeier WW, Kelsey WP. Effects of reduced acid conditioning time on enamel microleakage. Gen Dent 1987;35(4):278–80.
[5] Pashley DH, Carvalho RM, Sano H, et al. The microtensile bond test: a review. J Adhes Dent 1999;1(4):299–309.

[6] Miranda C, Prates LH, Vieira Rde S, et al. Shear bond strength of different adhesive systems to primary dentin and enamel. J Clin Pediatr Dent 2006;31(1):35–40.

[7] Kamada K, Yoshida K, Taira Y, et al. Shear bond strengths of four resin bonding systems to two silica-based machinable ceramic materials. Dent Mater J 2006;25(3):621–5.

[8] Arias VG, Ambrosano GMB, Pimneta LAF. Determination of the sample and plot size for microtensile testing [abstract 818]. J Dent Res 2006;85(spec issue A):85. Available at: http://iadr.com/publications/citingelectronic.html.

[9] Türkün SL. Clinical evaluation of a self-etching and a one-bottle adhesive system at two years. J Dent 2003;31(8):527–34.

[10] Di Renzo M, El Feninat F, Jiménez-Esquivel B, et al. Adhesion to dentin: the role of chemical reactions in surface modification. Can J Chem 1998;76(1):1–6.

[11] Moszner N, Salz U, Zimmerman J. Chemical aspects of self-etching enamel-dentin adhesives: a systematic review. Dent Mater 2005;21(10):895–910.

[12] Yavari M. Investigations of phosphatemediated adhesion to dentin surfaces. Montreal (Quebec, Canada): McGill University; 1999. p. 44–52.

[13] Yoshida Y, Van Meerbeek B, Nakayama Y, et al. Adhesion to and decalcification of hydroxyapatite by carboxylic acids. J Dent Res 2001;80(6):1565–9.

[14] Ten Cate AR. Oral histology: development, structure, and function. 5th edition. St. Louis (MO): Mosby-Year Book; 1998. p. 1.

[15] Di Renzo M, Ellis TH, Sacher E, et al. A photoacoustic FTIRS study of the chemical modifications of human dentin surfaces: I. Demineralization. Biomaterials 2001;22(8):787–92.

[16] Habelitz S, Marshall SJ, Marshall GW Jr, et al. Mechanical properties of human dental enamel on the nanometre scale. Arch Oral Biol 2001;46(2):173–83.

[17] Breschi L, Gobbi P, Mazzotti G, et al. Field emission in-lens SEM study of enamel and dentin. J Biomed Mater Res 1999;46(3):315–23.

[18] Thylstrup A, Leach SA, Qvist V, editors. Dentine and dentine reactions in the oral cavity. Oxford (UK): IRL Press, Ltd; 1987. p. 17–26.

[19] Ritter AV, Swift EJ Jr, Yamauchi M. Effects of phosphoric acid and glutaraldehyde-HEMA on dentin collagen. Eur J Oral Sci 2001;109(5):348–53.

[20] DiRenzo M, Ellis TH, Sacher E, et al. Adhesion to mineralized tissue: bonding to human dentin. Prog Surf Sci 1995;50(1):407–18.

[21] LeGeros RZ. Calcium phosphates in oral biology and medicine. Basel (Switzerland): Karger; 1991.

[22] Chahal O, Stangel I, Ellis T, et al. The effect of pH and acid anion of protein loss from dentin [abstract 2630]. J Dent Res 1996;75(special issue):346.

[23] Barkmeier WW, Erickson RL. Shear bond strength of composite to enamel and dentin using scotchbond multi-purpose. Am J Dent 1994;7(3):175–9.

[24] Pashley D, Tay FR. Aggressiveness of contemporary self-etching adhesives. Dent Mater 2001;17(5):430–44.

[25] Perdigao J, Geraldeli S. Bonding characteristics of self-etching adhesives to intact versus prepared enamel. J Esthet Restor Dent 2003;15(1):32–41.

[26] Perdigao J, Gomes G, Duarte S Jr, et al. Enamel bond strengths of pairs of adhesives from the same manufacturer. Oper Dent 2005;30(4):492–9.

[27] Miguez PA, Castro PS, Nunes MF, et al. Effect of acid-etching on the enamel bond of two self-etching systems. J Adhes Dent 2003;5(2):107–12.

[28] Torii Y, Itou K, Nishitani Y, et al. Effect of phosphoric acid etching prior to self-etching primer application on adhesion of resin composite to enamel and dentin. Am J Dent 2002;15(5):305–8.

[29] Van Landuyt KL, Peumans M, De Munck J, et al. Extension of a one-step self-etch adhesive into a multi-step adhesive. Dent Mater 2006;22(6):533–44.

[30] Lopes GC, Baratieri CM, Baratieri LN, et al. Bonding to cervical sclerotic dentin: effect of acid etching time. J Adhes Dent 2004;6(1):19–23.

[31] Di Renzo M, Ellis TH, Domingue A, et al. Chemical reactions between dentin and bonding agents. J Adhes 1994;47(1):115–21.

[32] Fukuda R, Yoshida Y, Nakayama Y, et al. Bonding efficacy of polyalkenoic acids to hydroxyapatite, enamel and dentin. Biomaterials 2003;24(11):1861–7.

[33] Inoue S, Abe Y, Yoshida Y, et al. Effect of conditioner on bond strength of glass-ionomer adhesive to dentin/enamel with and without smear layer interposition. Oper Dent 2004; 29(6):685–92.

[34] Yip HK, Tay FR, Ngo HC, et al. Bonding of contemporary glass ionomer cements to dentin. Dent Mater 2001;17(5):546–70.

[35] Nakabayashi N, Kojima K, Masuhara E. The promotion of adhesion by the infiltration of monomers into tooth substrate. J Biomed Mater Res 1982;16(3):265–73.

[36] Gwinnett AJ. Qualitative contribution of resin infiltration/hybridization to dentin bonding. Am J Dent 1993;6(1):7–9.

[37] Nakabayashi N, Nakamura M, Yasuda N. Hybrid layer as dentin-bonding mechanism. J Esthet Dent 1991;3(4):133–8.

[38] Gwinnett AJ, Tay FR, Pang KM, et al. Quantitative contribution of the collagen network in dentin hybridization. Am J Dent 1996;9(4):140–4.

[39] Prati C, Chersoni S, Pashley DH. Effect of removal of surface collagen fibril on resin-dentin bonding. Dent Mater 1999;15(5):323–31.

[40] Phrukkanon S, Burrow MF, Hartley PG, et al. The influence of the modification etched bovine dentin on bond strengths. Dent Mater 2000;16(4):255–65.

[41] Silva CH, Guenka Palma Dibb R, Sincler Delfino C, et al. Bonding performance of different adhesive systems to deproteinized dentin: microtensile bond strength and scanning electron microscopy. J Biomed Mater Res B Appl Biomater 2005;75(1):158–67.

[42] Abnar M, Farely EP. Potential use of organic polyphophonates as adhesives in the restoration of teeth. J Dent Res 1974;53:879–88.

[43] Munksgaard EC, Asmussen E. Bond strength between dentin and restorative resins mediated by mixtures of HEMA and glutaraldehyde. J Dent Res 1984;63:1087–9.

[44] Stangel I, Ostro E, Domingue A, et al. Photoacoustic fourier transform IR spectroscopic study of polymer-dentin interaction. In: Pireaux JJ, Bertrand P, Bredas JL, editors. An international conference on polymer-solid interfaces. Bristol (England): Institute of Physics Publishing; 1992. p. 157–67.

[45] Xu J, Stangel I, Butler IS, et al. An FT-Raman spectroscopic investigation of dentin and collagen surfaces modified by 2-hydroxyethylmethacrylate. J Dent Res 1997;76(1): 596–601.

[46] Asmussen E, Uno S. Adhesion of restorative resins to dentin: chemical and physicochemical aspects. Oper Dent 1992;(Suppl 5):68–74.

[47] Kugel G, Ferrari M. The science of bonding: from first to sixth generation. J Am Dent Assoc 2000;131(Suppl):20–5.

[48] Jacobsen T, Ma R, Soderholm KJ. Dentin bonding through interpenetrating network formation. Transactions of the Academy of Dental Materials 1994;7:45–52.

[49] Nakabayashi N, Takarada K. The effect of HEMA on bonding to dentin. Dent Mater 1992; 8(2):125–30.

[50] Fong W, Grunwald E. Acid dissociation in acetone-water mixtures: an anomalous medium effect when London dispersion forces are large. J Phys Chem 1969;73(11): 3909–12.

[51] Mohan B, Kandaswamy D. A confocal microscopic evaluation of resin-dentin interface using adhesive systems with three different solvents bonded to dry and moist dentin: an in vitro study. Quintessence Int 2005;36(7–8):511–21.

[52] Abate PF, Rodriguez VI, Macchi RL. Evaporation of solvent in one-bottle adhesives. J Dent 2000;28(6):437–40.

[53] Perdigao J, Swift EJ Jr, Lopes GC. Effects of repeated use on bond strengths of one-bottle adhesives. Quintessence Int 1999;30(12):819–23.

[54] Pashley DH, Agee KA, Nakajima M, et al. Solvent-induced dimensional changes in EDTA-demineralized dentin matrix. J Biomed Mater Res 2001;56(2):273–81.

[55] El Feninat F, Ellis TH, Sacher E, et al. A tapping mode AFM study of collapse and denaturation in dentinal collagen. Dent Mater 2001;17(4):284–8.

[56] El Feninat F, Ellis TH, Sacher E, et al. Moisture-dependent renaturation of collagen in phosphoric acid etched human dentin. J Biomed Mater Res 1998;42(4):549–53.

[57] Imazato S, McCabe JF, Tarumi H, et al. Degree of conversion of composites measured by DTA and FTIR. Dent Mater 2001;17(2):178–83.

[58] Van Meerbeek B, De Munck J, Yoshida Y, et al. Buonocore memorial lecture: adhesion to enamel and dentin. Current status and future challenges. Oper Dent 2003;28(3):215–35.

[59] Spencer P, Wang Y, Walker MP, et al. Interfacial chemistry of the dentin/adhesive bond. J Dent Res 2000;79(7):1458–63.

[60] Miyazaki M, Onose H, Moore BK. Analysis of the dentin-resin interface by use of laser Raman spectroscopy. Dent Mater 2002;18(8):576–80.

[61] Sano H, Shono T, Takatsu T, et al. Microporous dentin zone beneath resin-impregnated layer. Oper Dent 1994;19:59–64.

[62] Jacobsen T, Soderholm KJ. Some effects of water on dentin bonding. Dent Mater 1995; 11(2):132–6.

[63] Gregoire GL, Akon BA, Millas A. Interfacial micromorphological differences in hybrid layer formation between water- and solvent-based dentin bonding systems. J Prosthet Dent 2002;87(6):633–41.

[64] Salz U, Zimmermann J, Zeuner F, et al. Hydrolytic stability of self-etching adhesive systems. J Adhes Dent 2005;7(2):107–16.

[65] Pashley DH, Carvalho RM, Sano H, et al. The microtensile bond test: a review. J Adhes Dent 2001;1:299–309.

[66] Inoue S, Vargas MA, Abe Y, et al. Microtensile bond strength of eleven contemporary adhesives to dentin. J Adhes Dent 2001;3(3):237–45.

[67] Yap UJ, Stokes AN, Pearson GJ. Concepts of adhesion: a review. N Z Dent J 1994;90(401): 92–8.

[68] Peumans M, Kanumilli P, De Munck J, et al. Clinical effectiveness of contemporary adhesives: a systematic review of current clinical trials. Dent Mater 2005;21(9):864–81.

[69] Spencer P, Wang Y. Adhesive phase separation at the dentin interface under wet bonding conditions. J Biomed Mater Res 2002;62(3):447–56.

[70] Stangel I, Barolet RY. Clinical evaluation of two posterior composite resins: two-year results. J Oral Rehabil 1990;17(3):257–68.

[71] Ratih DN, Palamara JE, Messer HH. Dentinal fluid flow and cuspal displacement in response to resin composite restorative procedures. Dent Mater 2007 [Epub ahead of print].

[72] Casselli DS, Martins LR. Postoperative sensitivity in Class I composite resin restorations in vivo. J Adhes Dent 2006;8(1):53–8.

[73] Perdigao J, Geraldeli S, Hodges JS. Total-etch versus self-etch adhesive: effect on postoperative sensitivity. J Am Dent Assoc 2003;134(12):1621–9.

[74] Akpata ES, Behbehani J. Effect of bonding systems on post-operative sensitivity from posterior composites. Am J Dent 2006;19(3):151–4.

ELSEVIER
SAUNDERS

Dent Clin N Am 51 (2007) 695–712

THE DENTAL
CLINICS
OF NORTH AMERICA

Endodontic Materials

R. Scott Gatewood, DMD

Department of Endodontics, University of Mississippi School of Dentistry,
2500 North State Street, Jackson, MS 39216, USA

Current endodontic materials include those that have been thoroughly tested by scientific investigation, clinical usage, and time, as well as others that are the result of new knowledge in the field of dental materials. Knowing the particular qualities of materials can aid the clinician in choosing those that are appropriate for a given situation. Conversely, knowing the outcomes of clinical usage of materials can aid research into developing new and better endodontic materials. This continuum of research, development, use, and outcomes gives promise of new materials to meet existing needs.

Obturation materials

Gutta percha

Gutta percha is the most common root filling material in use today. This is interesting, because it is one of the oldest dental materials currently being used. The history of gutta percha goes back much earlier than its introduction into dentistry in the late nineteenth century. It is thought that in a 1656 book, John Trandescant, an Englishman, was referring to gutta percha when he wrote about "mazer wood," a pliable material that could be warmed in water and formed to different shapes [1].

In 1843, Dr. Jose D'Almeida of Singapore presented specimens called gutta percha to the Royal Asiatic Society of England. This rediscovery of gutta percha, with its property of being pliable when warmed and of stable dimensions in cool water, led it to be used as the first successful insulation material for underwater telegraph lines in 1848 [1]. The 1850s found gutta percha being used for an amazing array of items, including thread, surgical instruments, garments, gloves, pipes, pillows, maps, tents, and carpets. Golf balls made of gutta percha were widely used and referred to as "gutties" until the 1920s.

E-mail address: rgatewood@sod.umsmed.edu

0011-8532/07/$ - see front matter © 2007 Published by Elsevier Inc.
doi:10.1016/j.cden.2007.04.005

dental.theclinics.com

The fascination with gutta percha in manufacturing was short-lived, in part because of the property that made it popular initially. Its plasticity at slightly elevated temperatures allowed it to be formed into a myriad of products, but they lacked dimensional stability with changes in temperature. Also, vulcanization of rubber, a natural isomer of gutta percha, gave a product of considerably more dimensional stability, and a usable alternative to gutta percha. Only its use in golf balls and in dentistry survived into the twentieth century.

The introduction of gutta percha into dentistry is credited to Dr. Asa Hill, a Connecticut dentist. As a result of a search for a plastic restorative material, he produced a mixture of gutta percha and carbonate of lime and quartz as "Hill's Stopping" in 1847 [2]. It became a widely used restorative material. In 1867, Dr. G.A. Bowman reported using gutta percha to fill root canals. By 1887, S.S. White was manufacturing gutta percha points.

Gutta percha is produced from the juice of trees of the sapodilla family, which are indigenous to Malaysia, Indonesia, and Brazil. Natural rubber and gutta percha are polymers of the same monomer, isoprene (C_5H_8), with rubber being the cis isomer and gutta percha the trans isomer (Fig. 1). In 1942, C.W. Bunn reported that the crystalline phase of gutta percha could exist in two forms: (1) alpha phase, and (2) beta phase [1]. The alpha phase is the naturally occurring form of gutta percha from the tree. If this is heated above 65°C, it melts into an amorphous form. If the

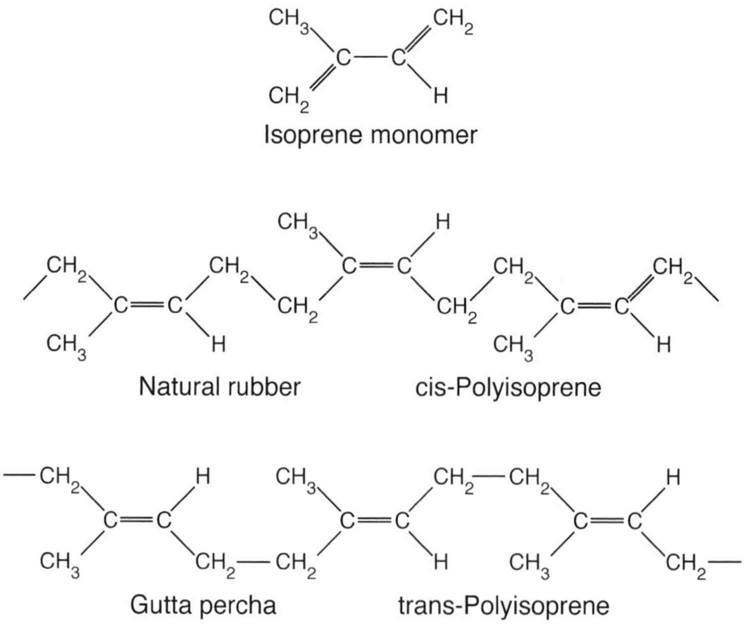

Fig. 1. Isomers of isoprene.

amorphous material is cooled very slowly (0.5°C per hour) it recrystallizes into the alpha phase. If the amorphous material is cooled faster, it recrystallizes as the beta phase.

The beta phase of gutta percha is used in commercially prepared dental gutta percha for endodontic use. By weight, dental gutta percha contains only about 20% gutta percha. Zinc oxide comprises about 75% of dental gutta percha. The remaining components are various combinations of metal sulfates (for radiopacity) along with waxes and resins [3]. The precise percentages of the components of a company's dental gutta percha are usually proprietary secrets, but as a group, dental gutta percha is about one fourth organic (gutta percha, waxes, resins) and three fourths inorganic (zinc oxide, metal sulfates).

Gutta percha cones are usually supplied by the manufacturer after having been sterilized by irradiation. For chairside sterilization, cones can be placed in 5.25% sodium hypochlorate (NaOCl) for 1 minute [4]. Gutta percha can be dissolved by organic solvents such as chloroform, halothane, and xylene.

Gutta percha alone cannot hermetically seal a canal, because it has no adhesive qualities. It requires a sealer to provide a seal of the canal-gutta percha interface. Gutta percha is often applied to a canal with some type of condensation pressure. This may be with a lateral condensing force applied with a spreader, or a vertical condensing force applied with a plugger. Both methods are designed to give better adaptation of gutta percha to the anatomic intricacies of the canal system; however, it has been shown that gutta percha cannot be truly compressed, but is compacted when pressure is applied [5].

Prolonged storage of gutta percha cones results in the cones becoming brittle, especially if exposed to air, light, and elevated temperature. This is thought to be caused by oxidation of the cones, and possibly from conversion of the beta crystalline phase to the naturally occurring alpha crystalline phase [6]. Refrigeration of gutta percha can extend the shelf life.

The biocompatibility of gutta percha has been thoroughly tested through cytotoxicity, mutagenicity, implantation, and usage tests [7–12]. The tests proved gutta percha to be biocompatible as a root filling material. In comparison to endodontic sealers, gutta percha shows less toxicity.

Resilon

Recently, a new material has been introduced that brings dentin bonding technology to root canal obturation. The principle of chemically bonding the root-filling material to the canal wall appears to have great potential for improving both the apical and coronal seal of the canal.

Resilon (Resilon Research, LLC, Madison, Connecticut) is a thermoplastic synthetic polymer based on polymers of polyester containing bioactive glass and radiopaque fillers [13]. The filler content is approximately 65%

by weight. Resilon handles like gutta percha, and is available in the same variety of master cones and accessory cones. Also, Resilon pellets are available to use in backfilling with thermoplasticized techniques. Thus, Resilon can be used in the same obturation techniques as gutta percha. The sealer used with Resilon is Epiphany Root Canal Sealant (Pentron Clinical Technologies, Wallingford, Connecticut). It is a dual-curable dentin resin composite sealer. The matrix is a mixture of ethoxylated glycidylmethacrylate and Bisphenol A epoxy (Bis-GMA), urethane dimethacrylate (UDMA), and hydrophilic difunctional methacrylates. The total filler content is about 70% by weight, and is composed of calcium hydroxide, barium sulfate, barium glass, and silica. A canal filled with this system is said to create a "mono-block" [13], in which the Resilon bonds to the Epiphany sealer, which in turn bonds to the dentin wall.

As with other dentin bonding systems, etching and priming of the dentin surface is required to achieve a chemical bond. Instructions for using the Resilon system include rinsing with 17% ethylenediaminetetraacetic acid (EDTA) to remove the smear layer, followed by Epiphany Primer, a self-etch primer containing sulfonic acid terminated functional monomer, hydroxethyl methacrylate (HEMA), water, and polymerization initiator. Then, the Epiphany Root Canal Sealant is applied to the canal followed by the Resilon core. After the canal is obturated, light curing for 40 seconds will cure the coronal 2 mm of the canal, and self-curing of the remainder of the canal will occur in 15 to 30 minutes [13]. Retreatment of Resilon-filled canals is possible, because the material can be softened and dissolved by chloroform.

Some in vitro tests [13,14] have shown the Resilon system superior to gutta percha/sealer in leakage testing, whereas others [15,16] have shown no significant difference. In a dog model, Shipper and colleagues [17] found less apical periodontitis associated with teeth filled with the Resilon system than those filled with gutta percha/sealer. An in vitro test [18] showed increased resistance to fracture for teeth filled with the Resilon system compared with those filled with standard gutta percha techniques.

Some concern has been raised regarding the potential for alkaline [19] or enzymatic [20] hydrolysis of the polymer in Resilon, and the success of dentinal bonding in the confines of the root canal system [21,22]. These and other in vitro and clinical usage and success studies are sure to be evaluated for this obturation system.

Sealers

To provide a fluid-tight seal of the canal space, a sealer is required along with the core obturating material. Because of this, the sealer has as much or more importance than the core material in providing a successful clinical outcome. Grossman [23] described a number of properties that would be found in an ideal sealer. Although no sealer possesses all these properties, some have more than others. Grossman's criteria are outlined in Table 1.

Table 1
Properties of and criteria for an ideal sealer

Properties	Criteria
Should be tacky when mixed to provide good adhesion between it and the canal wall when set.	The sealer should adhere to the obturating material, usually gutta percha, when placed in the canal, and should adhere to the canal wall with its irregularities to completely fill the canal space.
Should make a hermetic seal.	The core material itself does not provide an adhesive seal to the canal wall. To create and maintain a fluid-tight seal of the canal is a prime requirement of a sealer.
Should be radiopaque.	The sealer should contribute to the radiopacity of the root filling for visualization on radiographs and evaluation of obturation of lateral canals and apical ramifications.
Should not shrink upon setting.	Any shrinkage of the sealer would tend to create gaps at the dentin interface or within the core material, compromising the seal.
Should not stain tooth structure.	Components of sealer should not leach into dentin leading to coronal or cervical discoloration of the crown.
Should be bacteriostatic, or at least not encourage bacterial growth.	This property is desirable, but increasing the antibacterial qualities of a sealer also increases its toxicity to host tissues.
Should set slowly.	A sealer must have ample working time to allow for placement during obturation and adjustment in the case of immediate post-space preparation.
Should be insoluble in tissue fluids.	Stability of sealer when set is a prime factor in maintaining a hermetic seal over time. This is compromised if fluid contact causes dissolution of the sealer.
Should be tissue-tolerant.	Biocompatibility of the sealer promotes periradicular repair. Most sealers tend to be more tissue-toxic in the unset state and considerably less toxic when fully set.
Should be soluble in a common solvent.	To allow for retreatment or post-space preparation, the sealer and the core material should be removable. This can be facilitated by using a solvent.

Data from Grossman L. Endodontic practice. 11th edition. Philadelphia: Lea and Febiger; 1988. p. 255.

Although no sealer meets all properties of Grossman's ideal sealer, there are many sealers available that are clinically acceptable and widely used. They can be classified into the general groups of zinc oxide-eugenol–based, polymers, calcium hydroxide-based, glass-ionomer, and resin-based.

Zinc oxide-eugenol–based sealers

These sealers have a long history of successful use, and have been the standard against which many newer sealers have been measured. Based on zinc oxide powder mixed with eugenol, numerous proprietary variations have been applied to these basic components to enhance various qualities of the sealer, such as dentin adhesion, reducing inflammation, or antibacterial action.

Grossman's formula (non-staining), introduced in 1958, is an industry standard for zinc oxide-eugenol sealers [24]. The components of the powder, listed below, are mixed with eugenol to form the sealer:

Zinc oxide 42%
Staybellite resin 27%
Bismuth subcarbonate 15%
Barium sulfate 15%
Sodium borate 1%

The resin component is added to increase the adhesive quality of the sealer. Also, the resin can react with zinc to produce a matrix-stabilized zincresinate that decreases the solubility of the sealer [25]. Barium sulfate increases radiopacity. The proportion of bismuth subcarbonate to sodium borate regulates the working and setting times of the sealer. A number of zinc oxide-eugenol sealers are variations from this original formula.

The setting reaction of the sealer is by formation of zinc eugenolate crystals embedded with zinc oxide. Free eugenol is present as the material sets and decreases as the setting process continues. It is the free eugenol that contributes most to the cytotoxicity of freshly mixed, unset sealer.

All zinc oxide-eugenol sealers have ample working time, but will set faster in the presence of body temperature and humidity than on a mixing slab. Smaller particle size of the zinc oxide component will increase the setting time. Longer and more vigorous spatulation while mixing will decrease setting time [26–28].

Calcium hydroxide-based sealers

Several sealers have been marketed that contain calcium hydroxide as part of a zinc oxide-eugenol or epoxy material. These sealers were developed with the idea of taking advantage of the biocompatibility and possible bioactivity of calcium hydroxide when placed adjacent to vital tissue in pulp caps or apexification; however, to be effective in this respect, calcium hydroxide must dissociate into calcium and hydroxyl ions. For this to occur, it would require the sealer to break down or dissolve to some degree. If dissolution of the calcium hydroxide component occurred, the likelihood of the sealing ability being compromised would increase.

There are no objective data to show that calcium hydroxide-based sealers possess the biologic effects associated with calcium hydroxide paste. The short-term sealing ability of the sealers has proved adequate [29,30], but questions about long-term stability remain [31].

Polymer-based sealers

Epoxy resins and a polyketone compound are examples of polymers used as endodontic sealers. The epoxy resin materials show good handling characteristics and adhesion to dentin [32], but significant toxicity in the unset state [11,33]. Interestingly, after 24 hours, the epoxy sealer has one of the lowest toxicities of endodontic sealers [34].

The polyketone sealer is a resin-reinforced chelate formed between zinc oxide and diketone [35]. The material has a tacky consistency, that while providing good adhesion to dentin, contributes to its somewhat difficult handling characteristics. The solubility is low [36], but cellular toxicity has been shown to be elevated [11,12,33].

Glass-ionomer sealers

Glass-ionomer sealer has the advantage of chemically bonding to dentin. This offers the potential of improving the seal and possibly strengthening the root against fracture. Some studies have shown that canals obturated using gutta percha with glass ionomer sealer were more resistant to fracture than when other sealers were used [37], whereas other studies showed no difference [38,39].

Glass-ionomer materials tend to show good biocompatibility [40]. The glass-ionomer sealer is viscous and has a shorter working time than many other sealers. Because of its hardness and relative insolubility in gutta percha solvents, retreatment can be more difficult [41].

Irrigation materials

Thorough irrigation of the canal system during instrumentation is an essential part of the process of rendering the canal system free of tissue, bacteria and bacterial products, and dentinal debris. This creates an environment favorable to successful obturation, and ultimately to clinical success.

Sterile saline

Sterile saline has been recommended by some as an endodontic irrigant. It has the advantage of biocompatibility over other irrigants, and Baker and colleagues [42] concluded through scanning electron microscope (SEM) evaluation that the type of irrigant used was not as important as the volume used in terms of removing canal debris. Using saline as an irrigant relies totally on the physical flushing action of irrigation to remove debris. It has none of the tissue-solvent or antibacterial effects that are beneficial in an endodontic irrigant.

Sodium hypochlorite

The most common endodontic irrigant for many years has been sodium hypochlorite (NaOCl). Its first reported use in modern medicine was in 1915, when Dakin [43] recommended a 0.5% solution of NaOCl for debridement of infected wounds.

NaOCl has a broad-spectrum antimicrobial effect, and is capable of killing bacteria, spores, fungi, and viruses. Concentrations varying from 1% to 5.25% are commonly used, and proponents of each concentration claim effective antimicrobial properties [44]. Used clinically, it is important to replenish NaOCl frequently, because its antimicrobial properties rely on free chlorine from dissociation of NaOCl, and this is what is consumed during tissue breakdown [45]. In small canals or canal ramifications, if NaOCl cannot contact the microbes, the antimicrobial effect is compromised. This is probably why in vivo antimicrobial tests of NaOCl do not always replicate in vitro results. In vitro studies have shown concentrations from 1% to 5% will kill any organism isolated from the root canal, but in vivo, the success of NaOCl depends on canal preparation to remove gross debris and to enlarge the canal so that the NaOCl can penetrate to the apical part of the canal.

NaOCl is usually supplied as a 5.25% solution. The tissue-solvent and antimicrobial effects are increased with elevated temperature, and Cunningham [46,47] found equal efficiency with 2.6% or 5.25% solutions at 37°C. The effectiveness also increases as the pH is decreased, but at pH less than 9, NaOCl becomes unstable and toxicity of vital tissue is increased [44]. For stability, commercially available NaOCl is buffered to a pH of 11 to 12.5.

Sodium hypochlorite is capable of dissolving tissue as well as the predentin layer of dentin. Some studies have shown better necrotic tissue solvent effects with 5.25% concentrations [48], whereas others show no difference with concentrations down to 1% [49]. Time of usage and contact time play a part in the solvent effects of NaOCl, so in the clinical setting with NaOCl in the canals for upwards of an hour, it is likely the lower concentrations perform acceptably. Gutta percha cones can be decontaminated by soaking for 1 minute in 1% NaOCl, or for 5 minutes in 0.5% [50].

Irrigation with NaOCl must be done with care not to inject the solution past the apical foramen into the periradicular tissues. The caustic effects of NaOCl in such an incident are manifested with severe pain, periapical bleeding, and almost immediate swelling [51,52]. Slow irrigation, light pressure, and use of a non-binding needle will prevent such an occurrence.

Chlorhexidine

Chlorhexidine gluconate, a bisguanide, is an antibacterial material that has attracted attention as an endodontic irrigant. Chlorhexidine in a 0.2% solution has been widely used as an oral rinse for plaque control, whereas a 2% solution is more commonly used as an endodontic irrigant. The antibacterial quality of chlorhexidine raises its potential as an irrigant, but it has no ability to dissolve tissue remnants as NaOCl does. This could contribute to a decreased overall cleaning ability of chlorhexidine when used during endodontic instrumentation. Yamashita and colleagues [53] found the use of 2% chlorhexidine resulted in inferior cleaning of canals when compared with 2.5% NaOCl or 2.5% NaOCl/EDTA. Clegg and coworkers [54], in an in vitro study, assessed the ability of chlorhexidine and various concentrations of NaOCl to disrupt a polymicrobial biofilm on hemisections of root apices. They found 2% chlorhexidine incapable of disrupting the biofilm, whereas 6%, 3%, 1% NaOCl and 1% NaOCl/MTAD disrupted the biofilm.

Chlorhexidine may not be suitable as a sole irrigant in endodontics, but may be a valuable adjunct to the use of NaOCl. Even though chlorhexidine is less effective against gram-negative than gram-positive bacteria [55], it is a gram-positive bacterium, *Enterococcus faecalis*, that is often found in persistent endodontic infections of previously root-filled teeth [56,57]. Dametto and colleagues [58] compared the antimicrobial activity of 2% chlorhexidine gel, 2% chlorhexidine liquid, and 5.25% NaOCl against *E faecalis*-infected canals immediately after instrumentation and 7 days after instrumentation. The chlorhexidine gel and liquid were significantly more effective than NaOCl in maintaining low colony forming units of *E faecalis* at 7 days. Oncag and coworkers [59] also found more residual antibacterial effects for 2% chlorhexidine than for NaOCl. This effect could be caused by the affinity of chlorhexidine to dental hard tissues leading to a persistent antibacterial action [60]. Because of this dentin affinity and the efficacy of chlorhexidine against *E faecalis*, Zehnder [61] and Stuart and colleagues [62] have suggested using chlorhexidine as a final rinse after canal instrumentation with NaOCl or as an intracanal medicament.

Smear layer removal

During instrumentation, a smear layer is formed along the canal wall. The smear layer, from 1 to 2 μm thick [63], contains organic and inorganic components from the cutting and scraping action of the files in the canal. Bacteria, if present, may also be part of the smear layer. A debate continues regarding the necessity of removing the smear layer. Removing it allows potentially better adaptation of the sealer to the dentin wall, and could improve sealer adhesion and the seal of the canal. Leaving the smear layer could decrease the permeability of dentin to future leakage. Evidence and opinions remain divided on this issue [64–66].

Ethylenediaminetetraacetic acid

EDTA is a chelating material that is capable, when used with NaOCl, of removing the smear layer. Sodium hypochlorite is needed to dissolve the organic components of the smear layer [67]. Following with EDTA irrigation will remove the inorganic portion of the smear layer and increase the diameter of the dentinal tubules [68]. A 17% solution of EDTA is normally used in endodontics, and is capable of removing the smear layer with 1 minute of contact time [45].

MTAD

Recently a material, MTAD (Biopure MTAD, Dentsply Tulsa Dental, Tulsa, Oklahoma), has been produced that proponents feel enhances and improves removal of the smear layer. MTAD is a mixture of 3% doxycycline, 4.25% citric acid, and 0.5% Tween-80, a polysorbate-80 detergent [69]. When used as a final rinse after using NaOCl as an irrigant during canal instrumentation, MTAD resulted in complete removal of the smear layer without significant change to the structure of dentinal tubules [70]. When compared with EDTA, MTAD showed significantly cleaner dentinal tubules in the apical one third, and significantly less erosion of dentinal tubules [69].

The antibacterial qualities of MTAD have been tested with various results. An in vitro study showed that MTAD was as effective as 5.25% NaOCl and more effective than EDTA in killing *E faecalis* [71], whereas another study showed no difference in antimicrobial efficacy for irrigation with 5.25% NaOCl/15% EDTA versus irrigation with 1.3% NaOCl/MTAD in the apical 5 mm of roots infected with *E faecalis* [72]. For antifungal efficacy, NaOCl and chlorhexidine were shown to be significantly superior to MTAD or EDTA [73].

In an evaluation of the cytotoxicity of MTAD and other endodontic materials using L929 fibroblasts, MTAD was less cytotoxic than eugenol, 3% H_2O_2, $Ca(OH)_2$ paste, 5.25% NaOCl, chlorhexidine, and EDTA, and more cytotoxic than 2.63%, 1.31%, and 0.66% NaOCl [74]. A recent in vitro study showed red-purple staining of light-exposed dentin when canals were rinsed with 1.3% NaOCl followed by MTAD [75]. It is thought that the staining resulted from photo-oxidation of the tetracycline in MTAD, giving a reddish-purple degradation product that binds to hydroxyapatite in dentin. Tay and colleagues [75] suggest the discoloration may be prevented by rinsing with ascorbic acid before MTAD.

Root-end filling materials

Surgical root canal therapy is often the indicated treatment when nonsurgical retreatment has failed or cannot be performed. Surgical root canal therapy usually involves resecting a portion of the root apex and preparing and filling a cavity preparation in the root end. The purpose of the retrograde filling is to seal the canal in order to prevent passage of bacteria or their toxins from the canal space into periradicular tissues. Practically every restorative material used on the crowns of teeth has been tried as a root-end filling material.

Amalgam

For many years, amalgam was the most commonly used retrograde filling material. It provided an acceptable apical seal and functioned in the periapical environment. Over time, studies began to suggest that other materials might replace amalgam as the retrograde filling material of choice. Such factors as the effects of mercury in the periapical tissues [76], leakage of amalgam retrofils [77,78], and concern about corrosion products [79] led to a search for alternative root-end filling materials.

Zinc oxide-eugenol

In a retrospective success study, Dorn and Gartner [80] compared amalgam with two reinforced zinc oxide-eugenol materials, IRM (L.D. Caulk Co., Milford, Delaware) and Super EBA (Harry J. Bosworth Co., Skokie, Illinois) as retrograde filling materials. Their results showed significantly higher success with IRM or Super EBA than with amalgam. The use of IRM and Super EBA as root-end filling materials began to increase, and continues to be popular among many practitioners. As is true of most zinc oxide-eugenol based materials, IRM and Super EBA show good results in leakage studies [81–84]. Because both materials contain eugenol in the liquid, the biocompatibility of the freshly set material could be questioned. Although this may be an issue in the short term, studies [76,85,86] suggest acceptable long-term biocompatibility for both materials.

Mineral trioxide aggregate

At Loma Linda University in the mid 1990s, a material was developed that has found numerous uses in endodontics, including as a root-end filling material. Mineral trioxide aggregate or MTA (ProRoot MTA, Dentsply Tulsa Dental) is composed primarily of tricalcium silicate, tricalcium aluminate, tricalcium oxide, and silicate oxide [87]. The material is 75% Portland cement. It sets in the presence of moisture, and has a hardening time of 2 hours 45 minutes to 4 hours.

Torabinejad [88,89] led the development and testing of the material to assess its suitability for use in dentistry. Numerous tests were done to evaluate the physical properties of MTA and its biocompatibility. In leakage tests, MTA showed significantly less leakage than amalgam, Super EBA, or IRM. Another study [90] measured the amount of time needed for *Staphylococcus aureus* to penetrate around 3-mm thickness of root-end fillings of amalgam, IRM, Super EBA, or MTA. MTA gave significantly less leakage than the other materials. The marginal adaptation of MTA and other root-end filling materials to the confines of a root-end cavity preparation was evaluated using an SEM [91]. MTA gave less marginal gap formation and better adaptation than amalgam, IRM, or Super EBA.

Studies in vitro and in vivo have supported the biocompatibility of MTA [87,92]. In a histologic study comparing MTA and amalgam as root-end fillings in monkeys, five of six root ends filled with MTA had a complete layer of cementum over the filling [93]. All root ends filled with amalgam showed periradicular inflammation with no cementum over the root-end filling material.

Because of its physical properties and biocompatibility, MTA has been used in numerous clinical situations besides as a root-end filling. It is used to repair perforations, to close open apices in apexification, as a direct pulp capping material, and to cover pulp stumps for apexogenesis.

In cases such as these, where the material must have a tissue interface, it has performed well. This could be in part because of the high pH of MTA, 10.2 initially and rising to 12.5 in 3 hours [94]. Additionally, Sarkar and coworkers [95] found that MTA exposed to synthetic tissue fluid at 37°C released its metallic constituents, primarily calcium, and produced precipitates with composition and structure similar to hydroxyapatite. They attribute the sealing ability, biocompatibility, and dentinogenic activity of MTA to this physiochemical reaction.

Intracanal medicaments

Thorough biomechanical cleaning of the root canal system is an accepted principle of endodontic therapy. This commonly involves the use of an antibacterial irrigant to help eliminate microorganisms from the canal. Even so, canals of teeth with nonvital pulps frequently retain viable bacteria after instrumentation [96,97]. To lower the bacterial count in such canals when treating in more than one appointment, various materials have been used between appointments as intracanal medicaments.

Volatile medicaments

Historically, as more emphasis was placed on the thoroughness of instrumentation and irrigation, less emphasis was placed on traditional volatile chemicals used as intracanal medicaments between appointments. Materials such as metacresylacetate, camphorated monoparachlorophenaol (CMCP), and formocresol show moderate to strong antibacterial qualities in vitro, but the empiric belief in their clinical usefulness has not been demonstrated. The duration of action of such materials when sealed in a tooth is short-lived [98,99]. Also, the toxicity of these volatile phenolics and aldehydes to vital tissue has been shown [100], as has the potential distribution of the materials into the body [101].

Calcium hydroxide

Currently, the material with the most scientific and popular support for use as an intracanal medicament is calcium hydroxide. Calcium hydroxide has been used in dentistry for over 60 years in a variety of applications such as pulp capping and apexification. When used as an intracanal medicament, calcium hydroxide powder can be mixed with sterile water, saline, or anesthetic, or a commercial preparation of calcium hydroxide can be used.

The pH of a calcium hydroxide/saline solution is reported as 12.5 [102], and it is thought that the high pH of the solution contributes to its antibacterial and biologic activities. The biocompatibility of calcium hydroxide is supported by its history of use as a pulp capping or apexification material. The antibacterial qualities of calcium hydroxide have been shown in a number of clinical studies [103–105]. Shuping and colleagues [105] showed a significant reduction of bacteria from canals instrumented using NaOCl irrigant followed by placement of calcium hydroxide for at least 1 week, when compared with canals instrumented in the same manner but without placement of calcium hydroxide. Because calcium hydroxide is not volatile and is usually placed in the canal in a pastelike consistency, its antibacterial action can be prolonged.

Wadachi and coworkers [106] showed calcium hydroxide to be an effective agent in removing tissue debris remaining on canal walls. Using extracted bovine incisors, soft tissue debris on canal walls was reduced remarkably in groups treated with 6% NaOCl for over 30 seconds or with calcium hydroxide for 7 days. The combination of calcium hydroxide treatment followed by NaOCl was more effective than the individual treatments alone. This evidence suggests the usefulness of calcium hydroxide in creating a canal as free as possible of bacteria and tissue debris.

Lipopolysaccharide (endotoxin) is a macromolecule found in the outer membrane of the cell wall of gram-negative bacteria, and is shed upon bacterial cell death. Many inflammatory responses are attributed to lipopolysaccharide, such as toxicity, pyrogenicity, macrophage activation, and complement activation [107]. Safavi and Nichols [108] found that calcium hydroxide could hydrolyze the lipid component of lipopolysaccharide, and suggested that by thus degrading its inflammatory potential, this could be an important reason for beneficial use of calcium hydroxide as an intracanal medicament.

Using a dog model, Katebzadek and colleagues [109] compared periapical healing after obturation of infected root canals, either in one appointment or after 1 week of calcium hydroxide treatment. Saline was the irrigant for both groups. They found calcium hydroxide treatment for 1 week before obturation gave superior results compared with one-step treatment. Trope and coworkers [110] reported a human study evaluating radiographic healing of teeth with apical periodontitis that were treated in one visit or two visits, with or without calcium hydroxide as an intracanal medicament. The periapical status was most improved in the calcium hydroxide group.

Summary

The biologic principles of endodontic therapy have been well-established. Thorough cleaning of the canal system to render it as free as possible of tissue, bacteria, and bacterial products, followed by complete obturation of the canal system to prevent apical or coronal leakage will create an environment that promotes periradicular healing. Different materials are available to achieve this objective, some having been used for over 100 years, whereas others are relatively new to the endodontic armamentarium. Ongoing efforts to improve the outcome of endodontic therapy will drive the continued development of new materials.

References

[1] Goodman A, Schilder H, Aldrich W. The thermomechanical properties of gutta percha. II. The history and chemistry of gutta percha. Oral Surg Oral Med Oral Pathol 1974;37(6): 954–61.

[2] Gutman JL, Milas VB. History. In: Cohen S, Burns RC, editors. Pathways of the pulp. 3rd edition. St. Louis (MO): The C.V. Mosby Company; 1984. p. 823–42.

[3] Friedman CE, Sandik JL, Heuer MA, et al. Composition and physical properties of gutta percha endodontic filling materials. J Endod 1977;3(8):304–8.

[4] Senia ES, Marraro RV, Mitchell JL, et al. Rapid sterilization of gutta percha cones with 5.25% sodium hypochlorite. J Endod 1975;1(4):136–40.

[5] Schilder H, Goodman A, Aldrich W. The thermomechanical properties of gutta percha. III. Determination of phase transition temperatures for gutta percha. Oral Surg Oral Med Oral Pathol 1974;38(1):109–14.

[6] Oliet S, Sorin SM. Effect of aging on the mechanical properties of hand-rolled gutta percha endodontic cones. Oral Surg Oral Med Oral Pathol 1977;43(6):954–62.

[7] Feldman G, Nyborg H. Tissue reaction to root filling materials. I. Comparison between gutta-percha and silver amalgam implanted in rabbit. Odontol Revy 1962;13:1.

[8] Mitchell DF. The irritational qualities of dental materials. J Am Dent Assoc 1959;59:954.

[9] Sjögren U, Sundqvist G, Nair PNR. Tissue reaction to gutta percha particles of various sizes when implanted subcutaneously in guinea pigs. Eur J Oral Sci 1995;103:313.

[10] Ha H. The effect of gutta percha, silver points and Rickert's root sealer on bone healing. J Can Dent Assoc 1957;23:385.

[11] Spångberg L. Biological effects of root canal filling materials. II. Effect in vitro of water-soluble components of root canal filling materials on HeLa cells. Odontol Revy 1969;20:133.

[12] Spångberg L. Biological effects of root canal filling materials. V. Toxic effect in vitro of root filling materials on HeLa cells and human skin fibroblasts. Odontol Revy 1969;20:427.

[13] Shipper G, Ørstavik D, Teixeira FB, et al. An evaluation of microbial leakage in roots filled with a thermoplastic synthetic polymer-based root canal filling material (Resilon). J Endod 2004;30(5):342–7.

[14] Tunga U, Bodrumlu E. Assessment of the sealing ability of a new root canal obturation material. J Endod 2006;32(9):876–8.

[15] Biggs SG, Knowles KI, Ibarrola JL, et al. In vitro assessment of the sealing ability of resilon/epiphany using fluid filtration. J Endod 2006;32(8):759–61.

[16] Pitout E, Oberholzer TG, Blignaut E, et al. Coronal leakage of teeth root-filled with gutta percha or resilon root canal filling material. J Endod 2006;32(9):879–81.

[17] Shipper G, Teixeira FB, Arnold RR, et al. Periapical inflammation after coronal microbial inoculation of dog roots filled with gutta-percha or resilon. J Endod 2005;31(2):91–6.

[18] Teixeira FB, Teixeira EC, Thompson JY, et al. Fracture resistance of roots endodontically treated with a new resin filling material. J Am Dent Assoc 2004;135(5):646–52.

[19] Tay FR, Pashley DH, Williams MC, et al. Susceptibility of a polycaprolactone-based root canal filling material to degradation. I. Alkaline hydrolysis. J Endod 2005;31(8):593–8.

[20] Tay FR, Pashley DH, Yiu CKY, et al. Susceptibility of a polycaprolactone-based root canal filling material to degradation. II. Gravimetric evaluation of enzymatic hydrolysis. J Endod 2005;31(10):737–41.

[21] Tay FR, Loushine RJ, Weller RN, et al. Untrastructural evaluation of the apical seal in roots filled with a polycaprolactone-based root canal filling material. J Endod 2005; 31(7):514–9.

[22] Tay FR, Loushine RJ, Lambrechts P, et al. Geometric factors affecting dentin bonding in root canal: a theoretical modeling approach. J Endod 2005;31(8):584–9.

[23] Grossman L. Endodontic practice. 11th edition. Philadelphia: Lea and Febiger; 1988. p. 255.

[24] Grossman L. Endodontic practice. 10th edition. Philadelphia: Lea and Febiger; 1982. p. 297.

[25] Matsuya Y, Matsuya S. Effect of abietic acid and polymethylmethacrylate on the dissolution process of zinc oxide-eugenol cement. Biomaterials 1994;15:307.

[26] Copeland HI, Brauer GM, Forziati A. The setting mechanism of zinc oxide and eugenol mixtures. J Dent Res 1955;34:740.

[27] Fragola A, Pascal S, Rosengarten M, et al. The effect of varying particle size of the components of Grossman's cement. J Endod 1979;5(11):336–9.

[28] Norman RD, Phillips RW, Swartz ML, et al. The effect of particle size on the physical properties of zinc oxide eugenol mixtures. J Dent Res 1964;43:252.

[29] Rothier A, Leonardo MR, Bonetti I, et al. Leakage evaluation in vitro of two calcium hydroxide and two zinc oxide-eugenol based sealers. J Endod 1987;13:336.

[30] Barnett F, Trope M, Rooney J, et al. In vivo sealing ability of calcium hydroxide-containing root canal sealers. Endod Dent Traumatol 1989;5:23.

[31] Tronstad L, Barnett F, Flax M. Solubility and biocompatibility of calcium hydroxide-containing root canal sealers. Endod Dent Traumatol 1988;4:152.

[32] Limkangwalmongkol S, Burscher P, Abbott PV, et al. A comparative study of the apical leakage of four root canal sealers and laterally condensed gutta percha. J Endod 1991;17: 495.

[33] Spångberg L. Biological effects of root canal filling materials. IV. Effect in vitro of solubilized root canal filling materials on HeLa cells. Odontol Revy 1969;20:289.

[34] Wennberg A, Ørstavik D. Adhesion of root canal sealers to bovine dentin and gutta percha. Int Endod J 1990;23:13.

[35] Ingle JI, Luebke RG, Zidell JD, et al. Obturation of the radicular space. In: Ingle JI, Taintor JF, editors. Endodontics. 3rd edition. Philadelphia: Lea and Febiger; 1985. p. 231.

[36] Higginbotham TL. A comparative study of the physical properties of five commonly used root canal sealers. Oral Surg Oral Med Oral Pathol 1967;24:89.

[37] Lertchirakarn V, Timyam A, Messer HH. Effects of root canal sealers on vertical root fracture resistance of endodontically treated teeth. J Endod 2002;28(3):212–9.

[38] Johnson ME, Stewart GP, Nielsen CJ, et al. Evaluation of root reinforcement of endodontically treated teeth. Oral Surg Oral Med Oral Pathol Oral Radiol Endod 2000;90(3): 360–4.

[39] Apicella MJ, Loushine RJ, Wesst LA, et al. A comparison of root fracture resistance using two root canal sealers. Int Endod J 1999;32(5):376–80.

[40] Zmener O, Dominquez FV. Tissue response to a glass ionomer used as an endodontic cement. Oral Surg Oral Med Oral Pathol 1983;56:198.

[41] Moshonov J, Trope M, Friedman S. Retreatment efficacy 3 months after obturation using glass ionomer cement, zinc oxide-eugenol, and epoxy resin sealers. J Endod 1994; 20:90.

[42] Baker NA, Eleazer PD, Averbach RE, et al. Scanning electron microscope study of the efficacy of various irrigating solutions. J Endod 1975;1(4):127–35.

[43] Dakin HD. On the use of certain antiseptic substances in treatment of infected wounds. Br Med J 1915;2:318.

[44] Mentz TCF. The use of sodium hypochlorite as a general endodontic medicament. Int Endod J 1982;15:132–6.

[45] Spångberg L. Instruments, materials, and devices. In: Cohen S, Burns RC, editors. Pathways of the pulp. 8th edition. St. Louis (MO): Mosby; 2002. p. 545–6.

[46] Cunningham WT, Balekjiam AY. Effect of temperature on collagen-dissolving ability of sodium hypochlorite endodontic irrigant. Oral Surg Oral Med Oral Pathol 1980;49:175.

[47] Cunningham WT, Joseph SW. Effect of temperature on the bactericidal action of sodium hypochlorite endodontic irrigant. Oral Surg Oral Med Oral Pathol 1980;50:569.

[48] Hand RE, Smith ML, Harrison JW. Analysis of the effect of dilution on the necrotic tissue dissolution property of sodium hypochlorite. J Endod 1978;4:60.

[49] Gordon TM, Damato D, Christner P. Solvent effect of various dilutions of sodium hypochlorite on vital and necrotic tissue. J Endod 1981;7:466.

[50] Cardoso C, Regiane-Kotaka C, Redmershi R, et al. Rapid decontamination of gutta percha cones with sodium hypochlorite. J Endod 1999;25:498–501.

[51] Becher GL, Cohen S, Borer R. The sequelae of accidentally injecting sodium hypochlorite beyond the root apex. Oral Surg Oral Med Oral Pathol 1974;38:633.

[52] Sabala CL, Powell SE. Sodium hypochlorite injection into periapical tissues. J Endod 1989; 15:490.

[53] Yamashita JC, Tanomaru FM, Leonardo MR, et al. Scanning electron microscopic study of the cleaning ability of chlorhexidine as a root-canal irrigant. Int Endod J 2003;36(6): 391–4.

[54] Clegg MS, Vertucci FJ, Walker C, et al. The effect of exposure to irrigant solutions on apical dentin biofilms in vitro. J Endod 2006;32(5):434–7.

[55] Emilson CG. Susceptibility of various microorganisms to chlorhexidine. Scand J Dent Res 1977;85:255–65.

[56] Sundqvist G, Figdor D, Persson S, et al. Microbiologic analysis of teeth with failed endodontic treatment and the outcome of conservative re-treatment. Oral Surg Oral Med Oral Pathol Oral Radiol Endod 1998;85:86–93.

[57] Peciuliene V, Balciuniene I, Eriksen H, et al. Isolation of *Enterococcus faecalis* in previously root-filled canals in a Lithuanian population. J Endod 2000;26:593–5.

[58] Dametto FR, Ferraz CC, de Almeida Gomes BP, et al. In vitro assessment of the immediate and prolonged antimicrobial action of chlorhexidine gel as an endodontic irrigant against *Enterococcus faecalis*. Oral Surg Oral Med Oral Pathol Oral Radiol Endod 2005;99(6): 768–72.

[59] Oncag O, Hosgor M, Hilmioglu S, et al. Comparison of antibacterial and toxic effects of various root canal irrigants. Int Endod J 2003;36(6):423–32.

[60] Parsons GJ, Patterson SS, Miller CH, et al. Uptake and release of chlorhexidine by bovine pulp and dentin specimens and their subsequent acquisition of antibacterial properties. Oral Surg Oral Med Oral Pathol 1980;49:455–9.

[61] Zehnder M. Root canal irrigants. J Endod 2006;32(5):389–98.

[62] Stuart CH, Schwartz SA, Beeson TJ, et al. *Enterococcus faecalis*: its role in root canal treatment failure and current concepts in retreatment. J Endod 2006;32(2):93–8.

[63] Mader CL, Baumgartner JC, Peters DD. Scanning electron microscopic investitgation of the smeared layer on root canal walls. J Endod 1984;10(10):477–83.

[64] Kennedy WA, Walker WA III, Gough RW. Smear layer removal effects on apical leakage. J Endod 1986;12(1):21.

[65] Madison S, Krell KV. Comparison of ethylenediamine tetraacetic acid and sodium hypochlorite on the apical seal of endodontically treated teeth. J Endod 1984;10(10): 499–503.

[66] Cooke HG, Grower MF, del Rio C. Effects of instrumentation with a chelating agent on the periapical seal of obturated root canals. J Endod 1976;2(10):312–4.

[67] Goldman M, Kunman JH, Goldman LB, et al. New method of irrigation during endodontic treatment. J Endod 1976;2:257.

[68] Goldberg F, Abramovich A. Analysis of the effect of EDTAC on the dentinal walls of the root canal. J Endod 1977;3(3):101–5.

[69] Torabinejad M, Khademi AA, Babagoli J, et al. A new solution for removal of the smear layer. J Endod 2003;29(3):170–5.

[70] Torabinejad M, Cho Y, Khademi AA, et al. The effect of various concentrations of sodium hypochlorite on the ability of MTAD to remove the smear layer. J Endod 2003;29(4):233–9.

[71] Torabinejad M, Shabahang S, Aprecio RM, et al. The antimicrobial effect of MTAD: an in vitro investigation. J Endod 2003;29(6):400–3.

[72] Kho P, Baumgartner JC. A comparison of the antimicrobial efficacy of NaOCl/Biopure MTAD verusu NaOCl/EDTA against *Enterococcus faecalis*. J Endod 2006;32(7):652–5.

[73] Ruff ML, McClanahan SB, Babel BS. In vitro antifungal efficacy of four irrigants as a final rinse. J Endod 2006;32(4):331–3.

[74] Zhang W, Torabinejad M, Li Y. Evaluation of cytotoxicity of MTAD using the MTT-tetrazolium method. J Endod 2003;29(10):654–7.

[75] Tay FR, Mazzoni A, Pashley DH, et al. Potential iatrogenic tetracycline staining of endodontically treated teeth via NaOCl/MTAD irrigation: a preliminary report. J Endod 2006; 32(4):354–8.

[76] Oynick J, Oynick T. A study of a new material for retrograde fillings. J Endod 1978;4:203–6.

[77] Kos WL, Aulozzi DP, Gerstein H. A comparative bacterial microleakage study of retrofilling materials. J Endod 1982;8:355–8.

[78] Abdal AK, Retief DH. The apical seal via the retrosurgical approach. I. A preliminary study. Oral Surg Oral Med Oral Pathol 1982;53:614–21.

[79] Ravenholt G. Corrosion current and pH rise around titanium coupled to dental alloys. Scand J Dent Res 1988;96:466–72.

[80] Dorn SO, Gartner AH. Retrograde filling materials: a retrospective success-failure study of amalgam, EBA, and IRM. J Endo 1990;16(8):391–3.

[81] Szeremeta-Brower TL, VanCura JE, Zaki AE. A comparison of the sealing properties of different retrograde techniques: an autoradiographic study. Oral Surg Oral Med Oral Pathol 1985;59:82–7.

[82] Beltes P, Zervas P, Lambrianidis T, et al. In vitro study of the sealing ability of four retrograde filling materials. Endod Dent Traumatol 1988;4:82–4.

[83] Smee G, Bolanos OR, Morse DR, et al. A comparative leakage study of P-30 resin bonded ceramic, teflon, amalgam, and IRM as retrofilling seals. J Endod 1987;13:117–21.

[84] Bondra DL, Hartwell GR, MacPherson MG, et al. Leakage in vitro with IRM, high copper amalgam, and EBA cement as retrofilling materials. J Endod 1989;15:152–60.

[85] Kearny WW. IRM: a tissue tolerance study [thesis]. Detroit (MI): University of Detroit; 1988.

[86] Blackman R, Gross M, Seltzer S. An evaluation of the biocompatibility of a glass ionomer-silver cement in rat connective tissue. J Endod 1989;15:76–9.

[87] Torabinejad M, Hong CU, Pitt Ford TR, et al. Tissue reaction to implanted super-EBA and mineral trioxide aggregate in the mandible of guinea pigs: a preliminary report. J Endod 1995;21(11):569–71.

[88] Torabinejad M, Watson TF, Pitt Ford TR. The sealing ability of a mineral trioxide aggregate as a root canal filling material. J Endod 1993;19:591–5.

[89] Torabinejad M, Higa RK, McKentry DJ, et al. Effects of blood contamination on dye leakage of root end filling materials. J Endod 1994;20:159–63.

[90] Torabinejad M, Falah Rastegar A, Kettering JD, et al. Bacterial leakage of mineral trioxide aggregate as a root end filling material. J Endod 1995;21:109–12.

[91] Torabinejad M, Wilder Smith P, Pitt Ford TR. Comparative investigation of marginal adaptation of mineral trioxide aggregate and other commonly used root end filling materials. J Endod 1995;21:295–9.

[92] Torabinejad M, Hong CU, Pitt Ford TR, et al. Cytotoxicity of four root end filling materials. J Endod 1995;21:489–92.

[93] Torabinejad M, Pitt Ford TR, McKendry DJ, et al. Histologic assessment of mineral trioxide aggregate as a root-end filling in monkeys. J Endod 1997;23(4):225–8.

[94] Torabinejad M, Hong CU, McDonald F, et al. Physical and chemical properties of a new root-end filling material. J Endod 1995;21(7):349–53.

[95] Sarkar NK, Caicedo R, Ritwik P, et al. Physiochemical basis of the biologic properties of mineral trioxide aggregate. J Endod 2005;31(2):97–100.

[96] Byström A, Sundqvist G. The antibacterial action of sodium hypochlorite and EDTA in 60 cases of endodontic therapy. Int Endod J 1985;18:35.

[97] McGurkin-Smith R, Trope M, Caplan D, et al. Reduction of intracanal bacteria using GT rotary instrumentation, 5.25% NaOCl, EDTA, and Ca(OH)$_2$. J Endod 2005;31(5):359–63.

[98] Messer H, Shepard C, Chen R-S. The duration of effectiveness of root canal medicaments. J Endod 1984;10:246.

[99] Fager FK, Messer HH. Systemic distribution of camphorated monochlorophenol from cotton pellets sealed in pulp chambers. J Endod 1986;12:225.

[100] Spångberg L, Engstrom G, Langeland K. Biologic effects of dental materials. III. Toxicity and antimicrobial effect of endodontic antiseptics in vitro. Oral Surg Oral Med Oral Pathol 1973;36:856.

[101] Hata G, Nishikawa I, Kawazoe S, et al. Systemic distribution of 14C-labeled formaldehyde applied in the root canal following pulpectomy. J Endod 1989;15:539.

[102] Stamos DG, Haasch GC, Gerstein H. The pH of local anesthetic/calcium hydroxide solutions. J Endod 1985;11(6):264–5.

[103] Byström A, Claesson R, Sundqvist G. The antimicrobial effect of camphorated paramonochlorophenol, camphorated phenol, and calcium hydroxide in the treatment of infected root canals. Endod Dent Traumatol 1985;1:170.

[104] Sjögren U, Figdor D, Spångberg L, et al. The antimicrobial effect of calcium hydroxide as a short-term intracanal dressing. Int Endod J 1991;24:119.

[105] Shuping GB, Orstavik D, Sigurdsson A, et al. Reduction of intracanal bacteria using nickel-titanium rotary instrumentation and various medications. J Endod 2000;26(12):751–5.

[106] Wadachi R, Araki K, Suda H. Effect of calcium hydroxide on the dissolution of soft tissue on the root canal wall. J Endod 1998;24(5):326–30.

[107] Morrison DC, Ryan JL. Endotoxins and disease mechanisms. Annu Rev Med 1987;38: 417–32.

[108] Safavi KE, Nichols FC. Effect of calcium hydroxide on bacterial lipopolysaccharide. J Endod 1993;19(2):76–8.

[109] Katebzadeh N, Sigurdsson A, Trope M. Radiographic evaluation of periapical healing after obturation of infected root canals: an in vivo study. Int Endod J 2000;33(1):60–6.

[110] Trope M, Delano EO, Orstavik D. Endodontic treatment of teeth with apical periodontitis: single vs. multivisit treatment. J Endod 1999;25(5):345–50.

ELSEVIER
SAUNDERS

Dent Clin N Am 51 (2007) 713–727

THE DENTAL
CLINICS
OF NORTH AMERICA

Recent Advances in Materials
for All-Ceramic Restorations

Jason A. Griggs, PhD

Department of Biomaterials Science, Baylor College of Dentistry, The Texas A & M
University System Health Science Center, 3302 Gaston Avenue, Dallas, TX 75246, USA

Ceramic materials are best able to mimic the appearance of natural teeth; however, two obstacles have limited the use of ceramics in the fabrication of dental prostheses: (1) brittleness leading to a lack of mechanical reliability, and (2) greater effort and time required for processing in comparison with metal alloys and dental composites. Recent advances in ceramic processing methods have simplified the work of the dental technician and have allowed greater quality control for ceramic materials, which has increased their mechanical reliability. As a result, the proportion of restorative treatments using all-ceramic prostheses is rapidly growing.

Several authors previously reviewed progress in the field of dental ceramics [1–12]. This article reviews the research literature and commercial changes over the past 3 years since the last review in this field. The recent developments in dental ceramic technology can be categorized into three primary trends:

There has been a rapid diversification of equipment and materials available for computer-aided design/computer-aided manufacturing (CAD-CAM) of ceramic prostheses.

The availability of CAD-CAM processing permitted the use of polycrystalline zirconia coping and framework materials. The relatively high stiffness and good mechanical reliability of partially stabilized zirconia allows thinner core layers, longer bridge spans, and the use of all-ceramic fixed partial dentures (FPDs) in posterior locations.

Basic science researchers are increasingly using clinically relevant specimen geometry, surface finish, and mechanical loading in their in vitro studies. This implies that in vitro results will more accurately predict clinical performance of ceramic prostheses; however, clinicians still need to be cautious in extrapolating from the laboratory to the clinical case.

E-mail address: jgriggs@bcd.tamhsc.edu

0011-8532/07/$ - see front matter © 2007 Elsevier Inc. All rights reserved.
doi:10.1016/j.cden.2007.04.006
dental.theclinics.com

Methods of ceramic fabrication

A recent review of the literature included a taxonomy of dental ceramics, in which materials were categorized according to their composition and indications [4]. The following sections are categorized by method of fabrication. This complements the previous review and reflects the recent diversification of CAD-CAM systems (Table 1). Ceramics having similar composition may be fabricated by different laboratory techniques, and each method of forming results in a different distribution of flaws, opportunity for depth of translucency, and accuracy of fit. These differences should be important to the clinician because they persist beyond the walls of the dental laboratory and affect clinical performance.

Powder condensation

This traditional method of forming ceramic prostheses involves applying a moist porcelain powder with an artist's brush, and removing excess moisture to compact the powder particles. The porcelain is further compacted by viscous flow of the glassy component during firing under vacuum. This method results in a large amount of residual porosity. The crystalline particles that strengthen the material on a microscopic scale are not connected to each other, but are separated by glassy regions. The porosity and discontinuous nature of the crystalline phase lead to relatively low strength and a wide variation in strength. Ceramics fabricated by powder condensation have greater translucency than can be achieved using other methods [13], so these materials are usually applied as the esthetic veneer layers on stronger cores and frameworks.

Slip casting

A slip is a low-viscosity slurry or mixture of ceramic powder particles suspended in a fluid (usually water). Slip casting involves forming a mold or negative replica of the desired framework geometry and pouring a slip into the mold. The mold is made of a material (usually gypsum) that extracts some water from the slip into the walls of the mold through capillary action, and some of the powder particles in the slip become compacted against the walls of the mold, forming a thin layer of green ceramic that is to become the framework. The remaining slip is discarded, and the framework can be removed from the mold after partial sintering, in order to improve the strength to a point where the framework can support its own weight. The resulting ceramic is very porous and must be either infiltrated with molten glass or fully sintered before veneering porcelain can be applied. Ceramics fabricated by slip casting can have higher fracture resistance than those produced by powder condensation, because the strengthening crystalline particles form a continuous network throughout the framework. Use of this method in dentistry has been limited to one series of three products for glass infiltration (In-Ceram, Vita Zahnfabrik, Bad Säckingen, Germany).

Table 1
Methods of forming ceramics for all-ceramic prostheses

Fabrication method	Commercial examples	Composition
Powder	Duceram LFC (Dentsply)[a]	Glass
condensation	Finesse Low Fusing (Dentsply)[a]	Leucite-glass
	IPS e.max Ceram (Ivoclar-Vivadent)[b]	Fluoroapatite-glass
	IPS Eris (Ivoclar-Vivadent)[b]	Fluoroapatite-glass
	LAVA Ceram (3M ESPE)[c]	Leucite-glass
	Vita D (Vita Zahnfabrik)[d]	Leucite-glass
	Vitadur Alpha (Vita Zahnfabrik)[d]	Leucite-glass
	Vitadur N (Vita Zahnfabrik)[d]	Alumina-glass
Slip casting	In-Ceram Alumina (Vita Zahnfabrik)[d]	Glass-alumina
	In-Ceram Spinell (Vita Zahnfabrik)[d]	Glass-alumina-spinel
	In-Ceram Zirconia (Vita Zahnfabrik)[d]	Glass-alumina-PS zirconia
Hot pressing	Finesse All-Ceramic (Dentsply)[a]	Leucite-glass
	Fortress Pressable (Mirage Dental Systems)[e]	Leucite-glass
	IPS Empress (Ivoclar-Vivadent)[b]	Lleucite-glass
	IPS Empress 2 (Ivoclar-Vivadent)[b]	Lithium disilicate-glass
	IPS e.max Press (Ivoclar-Vivadent)[b]	Lithium disilicate-glass
	IPS e.max ZirPress (Ivoclar-Vivadent)[b]	Fluoroapatite-glass
	OPC (Pentron Clinical Technologies)[f]	Leucite-glass
CAD-CAM		
Presintered	Cercon (Dentsply)[a]	Partially stabilized zirconia
	DC-Zirkon (DCS)[g]	Partially stabilized zirconia
	Everest ZS-Blanks (Kavo)[h]	Partially stabilized zirconia
	IPS e.max ZirCAD (Ivoclar-Vivadent)[b]	Partially stabilized zirconia
	LAVA Frame (3M ESPE)[c]	Partially stabilized zirconia
	Procera AllCeram (Nobel Biocare)[i]	Alumina
	Procera AllZirkon (Nobel Biocare)[i]	Partially stabilized zirconia
	Vita YZ (Vita Zahnfabrik)[d]	Partially stabilized zirconia
Densely sintered	Denzir (Cad.esthetics)[j]	Partially stabilized zirconia
	Digiceram L (Digident)[k]	Leucite-glass
	Digizon (Digident)[k]	Partially stabilized zirconia
	Everest G-Blanks (Kavo)[h]	Leucite-glass
	Everest ZH-Blanks (Kavo)[h]	Partially stabilized zirconia
	IPS e.max CAD (Ivoclar-Vivadent)[b]	Lithium disilicate-glass
	ProCAD (Ivoclar-Vivadent)[b]	Leucite-glass
	Vitablocs Mark II (Vita Zahnfabrik)[d]	Leucite-glass
	Vitablocs TriLuxe (Vita Zahnfabrik)[d]	Leucite-glass
	ZirKon (Cynovad)[l]	Partially stabilized zirconia
Glass infiltrated	In-Ceram Alumina (Vita Zahnfabrik)[d]	Glass-alumina
	In-Ceram Spinell (Vita Zahnfabrik)[d]	Glass-alumina-spinel
	In-Ceram Zirconia (Vita Zahnfabrik)[d]	Glass-alumina-PS zirconia

[a] York, Pennsylvania
[b] Schaan, Lichtenstein
[c] Saint Paul, Minnesota
[d] Bad Säckingen, Germany
[e] Kansas City, Kansas
[f] Wallingford, Connecticut
[g] Kelkheim, Germany
[h] Lake Zurich, Illinois
[i] Kloten, Switzerland
[j] Skellefteå, Sweden
[k] Pforzheim, Germany
[l] Saint-Laurent, Canada

The limited application of slip casting in dentistry is probably because the method requires a complicated series of steps, which provide a challenge to achieving accurate fit [14–16] and may result in internal defects that weaken the material from incomplete glass infiltration [17].

Hot pressing

The lost wax method is used to fabricate molds for pressable dental ceramics. Pressable ceramics are available from manufacturers as prefabricated ingots made of crystalline particles distributed throughout a glassy material. The microstructure is similar that of powder porcelains; however, pressable ceramics do not contain much porosity and can have a higher crystalline content, because the ingots are manufactured from nonporous glass ingots by applying a heat treatment that transforms some of the glass into crystals. This process can be expected to produce a well-controlled and homogeneous material. In the dental laboratory, the pressable ingots are heated to a temperature at which they become a highly viscous liquid, and they are slowly pressed into the lost wax mold. The advantage of hot pressing is that dental technicians are already experienced at achieving good accuracy of fit using the lost wax method with metal alloys [15,16]. Contrary to intuition, the higher crystalline content and lack of porosity do not lead to increased fracture resistance or decreased variability of strength [18]. Pressable ceramics usually have application only as core and framework materials. Pressable veneering materials, such as IPS e.max ZirPress (Ivoclar-Vivadent, Schaan, Liechtenstein) are available, but the depth of layered esthetics may be limited when using pressable ceramics for veneering materials.

Computer-aided design/computer-aided manufacturing

Like pressable ceramics, CAD-CAM ceramics are available as prefabricated ingots. These ingots are milled or cut by computer-controlled tools. In the case of presintered ceramics, the ingots are porous, which enables fast milling without bulk fracture of the ceramic. The disadvantage of presintered ingots is the need for subsequent sintering treatment to eliminate the porosity. The computer software must compensate for the shrinkage that occurs during sintering to achieve good accuracy of fit. Densely sintered ceramics are available in nonporous ingots, which are more difficult to mill, but they do not require any further sintering. Glass-infiltrated CAD-CAM ingots have similar composition to slip-cast ceramics, but starting with a porous ingot eliminates the complicated steps of slip casting. After milling, the porosity is eliminated by molten glass infiltration. One might question whether the milling process introduces surface cracks that weaken CAD-CAM ceramics, especially in the case of densely sintered ingots. An in vitro study confirmed the presence of such damage [19], and the in vivo studies reviewed later in this report suggest an effect on prosthesis longevity for inlays only. Dental CAD-CAM systems have been available for 20 years. In recent years, the increasing use of polycrystalline alumina and zirconia as framework materials and the increasing popularity and variety of CAD-CAM systems seem to be mutually accelerating trends.

Interpretation of in vitro reports

The results of in vitro tests reported in the scientific literature and in manufacturers' advertisements may not be predictive of clinical performance, so it is important for clinicians to be familiar with the following trends and to critically assess materials performance data.

There were 189 in vitro studies published from 2004 to 2006 on materials for all-ceramic prostheses (Table 2). The majority of studies pertained to comparison of mechanical reliability, marginal adaptation, or bonding to resin cements of commercially available materials, or the effects of varying fabrication protocols or surface treatments on these aspects of performance. Few studies were published regarding esthetic properties or the synthesis of novel ceramic compositions.

Most notably, there was a trend toward specimen geometry and loading conditions that better mimic the actual clinical situation. Many investigators have started testing multi-layered specimens with actual or simulated dentin, luting agent, core ceramic, and veneering ceramic layers. This is important because the surface treatments to prepare the core ceramic for application of the veneering ceramic have been shown to change the strength of the core ceramic [20], and the presence of the luting agent also has an effect on ceramic strength [21,22]. In addition, differential contraction of the core and veneering ceramics upon cooling creates thermally induced stresses, which alters the resistance of prostheses to stresses induced by mechanical loading [23]. It is also important to load specimens in a manner that reproduces the failure modes observed in the clinic. This includes blunt contact loading, cyclic fatigue loading, and loading in an aqueous environment [24], but reproducing all of these conditions does not guarantee

Table 2
Common topics for in vitro dental ceramic studies (2004–2006)

Method/topic of research	Number of studies[a]
Layered specimen geometry	70 (37%)
CAD-CAM fabrication	70 (37%)
Surface roughness/defects	57 (30%)
Cyclic mechanical/thermal loading	51 (27%)
Ceramic-resin bond strength	45 (24%)
Polycrystalline zirconia	33 (17%)
Marginal adaptation/degradation	24 (13%)
Contact loading	22 (12%)
Weibull statistics	22 (12%)
Polycrystalline alumina	11 (6%)

[a] Some studies were related to more than one of these methods/topics.

a clinically relevant failure mode. For example, a recent study on model glass-polymer systems showed that propagation of an "inner cone crack" from the contact surface results in bulk fracture of in vitro specimens [25], but analyses of clinically failed crowns show that bulk fracture originates from the core ceramic [26–28]. A noteworthy exception is that edge chipping originating from wear on contact surfaces has been observed clinically [29,30], and recent experiments with novel loading geometry have reproduced that failure mode in the laboratory [31,32]. There will always be a need for some simple standard geometry specimens to study the micromechanisms associated with crack growth; however, clinicians should not assume that simple specimens are predictive of clinical performance. In other words, ceramic specimens that have been finely polished, tested dry, or loaded quickly can be expected to have much higher strength than prostheses fabricated from the same materials, and the relative ranking of commercial products may change depending on test method.

An area that has seen only modest improvement is the reporting of Weibull statistics to describe ceramic strength data. The failure load and strength of a ceramic prosthesis or test specimen is controlled by the size of the largest flaw in the highly stressed location—not the average flaw. This causes the distribution of ceramic strengths to be skewed toward the lower end (Fig. 1). The strengths fit a Weibull distribution instead of a Gaussian (normal) distribution, and the shape of the Weibull distribution can be described by the Weibull modulus and the median strength (50% chance of failure) or the characteristic strength (63%). The Weibull modulus is a measure of variation in strength, with higher Weibull modulus corresponding to less variation. The Weibull modulus is more important than the median strength for predicting clinical performance, because the Weibull modulus can be used to predict the effect of prosthesis size on strength; it controls the stress levels

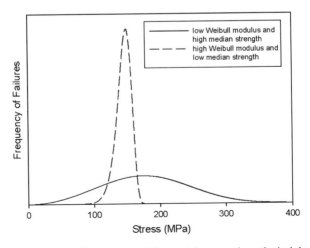

Fig. 1. Strength distributions for prostheses fabricated from two hypothetical dental ceramics.

corresponding to low probabilities of failure. The median strength corresponds to a 50% chance of failure, but clinicians are not interested in such a high failure rate. Fig. 2 illustrates how an all-ceramic system with lower median strength but higher Weibull modulus can survive higher stress levels at low probability of failure (5%). A slowly increasing number of basic science researchers are reporting Weibull statistics; however, they usually lack sufficient number of specimens to accurately estimate the Weibull modulus. Most studies published in the past 3 years used 6 to 10 specimens per group, even though the recommended number is 30 per group [33]. If a study estimates a Weibull modulus of m = 5 using a sample size of 10 specimens per group, then there is a 95% chance that the actual Weibull modulus for the restorative system is in the range of 3.7 to 9.2, and a 5% chance that the true value is outside that range [34]. Thus clinicians should be cautious, and note the sample size when interpreting in vitro studies, because a study may conclude that there is no difference in Weibull modulus between groups when there is not enough statistical power to detect a difference.

Survival of all-ceramic restorations

There were 35 clinical studies published from 2004 to 2006 on the longevity of all-ceramic restorations. It is important to analyze longevity data using Kaplan-Meier analysis [35], because simply dividing the number of failures observed by the total number of restorations placed results in artificially high reliability predictions [4]. Many of the reports did not provide sufficient details to perform the appropriate analysis, but those that did are separated here according to restoration type (veneer, inlay/onlay, crown, or FPD), and the cumulative survival probabilities are graphed in Figs. 3–6. Table 3 [36–55] summarizes the experimental factors for those studies.

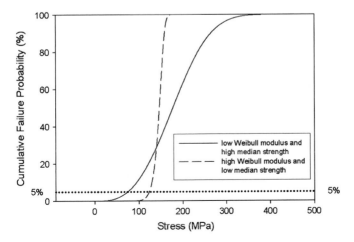

Fig. 2. Cumulative failure probabilities for prostheses fabricated from two hypothetical dental ceramics.

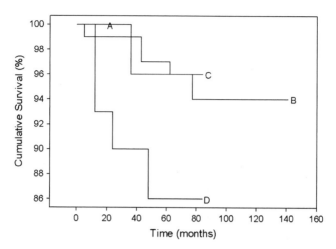

Fig. 3. Cumulative survival probabilities for all-ceramic veneers over time, calculated from data published in recent clinical studies.

Fig. 3 shows the survival of porcelain veneers over time. Groups C and D were part of a study to determine the effect of incisal porcelain on veneer longevity [48]. Group D veneers had no incisal porcelain and exhibited much shorter lifetimes than Group C veneers, which had incisal porcelain, and veneers from other studies. It is also noteworthy that the only groups with 100% short-term survival (36 months) were veneers with a layer of pressable ceramic.

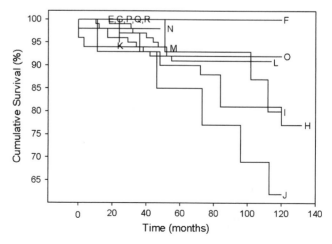

Fig. 4. Cumulative survival probabilities for all-ceramic inlays and onlays over time, calculated from data published in recent clinical studies.

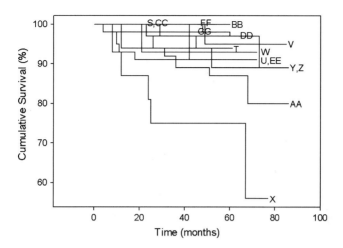

Fig. 5. Cumulative survival probabilities for all-ceramic crowns over time, calculated from data published in recent clinical studies.

Fig. 4 shows the survival of all-ceramic inlays and onlays over time. All of the groups have similar short-term survival. The most distinct trend is that long-term survival was related to ceramic fabrication method. The highest long-term survival probability (Groups F, L, M, N, and O) corresponded to inlays and onlays made from pressable ceramics. Groups H and I had the next highest long-term survival, and were both made from CAD-CAM ceramics. The lowest long-term survival probability (Group J) corresponded to inlays made by powder condensation.

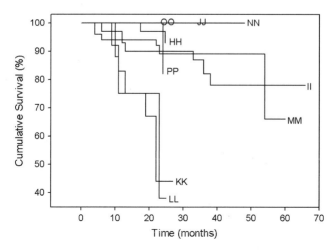

Fig. 6. Cumulative survival probabilities for all-ceramic fixed partial dentures over time, calculated from data published in recent clinical studies.

Table 3
Clinical studies reporting longevity of all-ceramic restorations

Graph label	Reference	Framework material	Veneer material	Luting agent	Restoration type	Location	Support
A	Barnes [36]	Finesse All-Ceramic	Finesse	DC	Veneer	Anterior	NS[a]
B	Fradeani [41]	IPS Empress	Vitadur Alpha	DC	Veneer	Anterior	NS
C	Smales [48]	Mirage	Mirage	DC	Veneer	Anterior	NS
D	Smales [48]	Mirage	none	DC	Veneer	Anterior	NS
E	Coelho Santos [39]	Duceram Plus	Duceram LFC	DC	Inlay	Posterior	NS
F	Coelho Santos [39]	IPS Empress	NS	DC	Inlay	Posterior	NS
G	Sjogren [47]	Vita Mark II	NS	SC	Inlay	Posterior	NS
H	Sjogren [47]	Vita Mark II	NS	DC	Inlay	Posterior	NS
I	Thordrup [51]	NS (CEREC)	NS	NS	Inlay	Posterior	NS
J	Thordrup [51]	Vitadur N	NS	NS	Inlay	Posterior	NS
K	Barnes [36]	Finesse Pressable	Finesse	DC	Inlay/onlay	Posterior	NS
L	Kramer [44]	IPS Empress	NS	NS	Inlay/onlay	Posterior	NS
M	Kramer [43]	IPS Empress	NS	DC, SE	Inlay/onlay	Posterior	NS
N	Kramer [43]	IPS Empress	NS	DC, ER	Inlay/onlay	Posterior	NS
O	Schulte [46]	IPS Empress	NS	LC	Inlay/onlay	Posterior	NS
P	Coelho Santos [39]	Duceram Plus	Duceram LFC	DC	Onlay	Posterior	NS
Q	Coelho Santos [39]	IPS Empress	NS	DC	Onlay	Posterior	NS
R	Kaytan [42]	IPS Empress	NS	DC	Onlay	Posterior	NS
S	Barnes [36]	Finesse Pressable	Finesse	DC	Single-unit crown	NS	NS
T	Bindl [37]	Vita Mark II	none	DC	Single-unit crown	Anterior	NS

U	Bindl [37]	In-Ceram Spinell	Vitadur Alpha	DC	Single-unit crown	Anterior	NS
V	Bindl [38]	Vita Mark II	NS	DC	Single-unit crown	Posterior	Classic premolar
W	Bindl [38]	Vita Mark II	NS	DC	Single-unit crown	Posterior	Reduced premolar
X	Bindl [38]	Vita Mark II	NS	DC	Single-unit crown	Posterior	Endo. premolar
Y	Bindl [38]	Vita Mark II	NS	DC	Single-unit crown	Posterior	Classic molar
Z	Bindl [38]	Vita Mark II	NS	DC	Single-unit crown	Posterior	Reduced molar
AA	Bindl [38]	Vita Mark II	NS	DC	Single-unit crown	Posterior	Endo. molar
BB	Marquardt [45]	IPS Empress 2	IPS Eris	DC	Single-unit crown	NS	NS
CC	Taskonak [50]	IPS Empress 2	NS	DC	Single-unit crown	NS	NS
DD	Walter [53]	Procera AllCeram	NS	GIC	Single-unit crown	Anterior	NS
EE	Walter [53]	Procera AllCeram	NS	GIC	Single-unit crown	Posterior	NS
FF	Zarone [55]	Procera AllCeram	NS	mod GIC	Single-unit crown	Anterior	Natural tooth
GG	Zarone [55]	Procera AllCeram	NS	mod GIC	Single-unit crown	Anterior	Implant
HH	Esquivel-Upshaw [40]	IPS Empress 2	NS	NS	Three-unit FPD	Posterior	NS
II	Marquardt [45]	IPS Empress 2	IPS Eris	DC	Three-unit FPD	NS	NS
JJ	Suarez [49]	In-Ceram Zirconia	NS	NS	Three-unit FPD	Posterior	NS
KK	Taskonak [50]	IPS Empress 2	NS	DC	Three-unit FPD	Anterior	NS
LL	Taskonak [50]	IPS Empress 2	NS	DC	Three-unit FPD	Posterior	NS
MM	Wolfart [54]	IPS e.max Press	stain	NS	Three-unit FPD	NS	NS
NN	Wolfart [54]	IPS e.max Press	stain	DC	Three-unit FPD	Posterior	NS
OO	Vult von Steyern [52]	DC-Zirkon	Vita D	ZP	Five-unit FPD	Anterior	NS
PP	Vult von Steyern [52]	DC-Zirkon	Vita D	ZP	Five-unit FPD	Posterior	NS

Abbreviations: ER, etch-and-rinse adhesive; DC, dual-cure resin cement; GIC, glass-ionomer cement; LC, light-cure resin cement; mod GIC, resin-modified glass-ionomer cement; SC, self-cure resin cement; SE, self-etch adhesive; ZP, zinc phosphate cement.

[a] NS indicates experimental factor was not specified or was not separated in the presentation of results.

Fig. 5 shows the survival of single-unit crowns over time. Groups X and AA showed much poorer longevity than the other groups. These crowns were part of a study to determine the effect tooth preparation on CAD-CAM crowns (Vita Mark II, Vita Zahnfabrik) [38]. Crowns in Groups V and Y were placed on teeth with sufficient healthy tissue for a classic crown preparation. Groups W and Z were placed on preparations with a reduced stump height. The shortest-lived crowns (Group X) were placed on end-odontically treated premolars, and the next shortest-lived crowns (Group AA) were placed on endodontically treated molars. Another interesting observation is that anterior crowns (Groups T and U) performed similarly to posterior crowns, even though lower biting forces, and hence longer prosthesis survival, are expected in the anterior.

Fig. 6 shows the survival of fixed partial dentures over time. The expected anterior-posterior relationship was observed here. Five-unit zirconia FPDs exhibited higher survival probability in anterior locations (Group OO) than in posterior locations (Group PP) [52]. Likewise, three-unit glass-ceramic FPDs exhibited higher survival probability in the anterior (Group KK) than the posterior (Group LL) [50]. This effect is not evident for another pressable glass-ceramic (Groups MM and NN), but it may have been con-founded by the other experimental factors, such as glass-ionomer cement in the anterior versus resin-based cement in the posterior. In fact, debonding was the primary cause of failure in that study [54]. The IPS Empress 2 FPDs (Group KK and LL) had a poor performance, because specimens in that study had smaller connector dimensions than recommended by the man-ufacturer (Burak Taskonak, DDS, PhD, personal communication, 2006).

Instead of ceramic fracture data, some studies reported survival in terms of percentage of restorations scoring "excellent" or "alpha" ratings at fol-low-up in each of the following categories: color match, marginal adapta-tion, marginal staining, secondary caries, and postoperative sensitivity. Most of those studies showed a lack of color match as the primary cause of low ratings at placement, and marginal deterioration (staining and lack of adaptation) as the primary problem at follow-up [36,41,42,56]. Hayashi and colleagues [57] collected more detailed observations on marginal deteri-oration than other investigators. They reported rapid wear of resin-based cements during the first 6 to 21 months, followed by a period of little change. At 72 months, inlay margins were widened by a rapid progression of ceramic microfractures.

References

[1] Anusavice KJ. Recent developments in restorative dental ceramics. J Am Dent Assoc 1993; 124(2):72–4, 76–8, 80–74.
[2] Deany IL. Recent advances in ceramics for dentistry. Crit Rev Oral Biol Med 1996;7(2): 134–43.

[3] Hayashi M, Wilson NH, Yeung CA, et al. Systematic review of ceramic inlays. Clin Oral Investig 2003;7(1):8–19.

[4] Kelly JR. Dental ceramics: current thinking and trends. Dent Clin North Am 2004;48(2): 513–30, viii.

[5] Kelly JR, Nishimura I, Campbell SD. Ceramics in dentistry: historical roots and current perspectives. J Prosthet Dent 1996;75(1):18–32.

[6] Martin N, Jedynakiewicz NM. Clinical performance of CEREC ceramic inlays: a systematic review. Dent Mater 1999;15(1):54–61.

[7] McLean JW. Evolution of dental ceramics in the twentieth century. J Prosthet Dent 2001; 85(1):61–6.

[8] Mormann WH, Bindl A. All-ceramic, chair-side computer-aided design/computer-aided machining restorations. Dent Clin North Am 2002;46(2):405–26, viii.

[9] Peumans M, Van Meerbeek B, Lambrechts P, et al. Porcelain veneers: a review of the literature. J Dent 2000;28(3):163–77.

[10] Piddock V, Qualtrough AJ. Dental ceramics—an update. J Dent 1990;18(5):227–35.

[11] Qualtrough AJ, Piddock V. Ceramics update. J Dent 1997;25(2):91–5.

[12] Raigrodski AJ. Contemporary all-ceramic fixed partial dentures: a review. Dent Clin North Am 2004;48(2):531–44, viii.

[13] Antonson SA, Anusavice KJ. Contrast ratio of veneering and core ceramics as a function of thickness. Int J Prosthodont 2001;14(4):316–20.

[14] Pallis K, Griggs JA, Woody RD, et al. Fracture resistance of three all-ceramic restorative systems for posterior applications. J Prosthet Dent 2004;91(6):561–9.

[15] Sulaiman F, Chai J, Jameson LM, et al. A comparison of the marginal fit of In-Ceram, IPS Empress, and Procera crowns. Int J Prosthodont 1997;10(5):478–84.

[16] Yeo IS, Yang JH, Lee JB. In vitro marginal fit of three all-ceramic crown systems. J Prosthet Dent 2003;90(5):459–64.

[17] Griggs JA, Taskonak B Jr, Mecholsky JJ Jr, et al. Reliability model for framework ceramic with multiple flaw populations. Orlando (FL): American Association for Dental Research; 2006.

[18] Tinschert J, Zwez D, Marx R, et al. Structural reliability of alumina-, feldspar-, leucite-, mica- and zirconia-based ceramics. J Dent 2000;28(7):529–35.

[19] Sindel J, Petschelt A, Grellner F, et al. Evaluation of subsurface damage in CAD/CAM machined dental ceramics. J Mater Sci Mater Med 1998;9(5):291–5.

[20] Carrier DD, Kelly JR. In-Ceram failure behavior and core-veneer interface quality as influenced by residual infiltration glass. J Prosthodont 1995;4(4):237–42.

[21] Fleming GJ, Maguire FR, Bhamra G, et al. The strengthening mechanism of resin cements on porcelain surfaces. J Dent Res 2006;85(3):272–6.

[22] Rosenstiel SF, Gupta PK, Van der Sluys RA, et al. Strength of a dental glass-ceramic after surface coating. Dent Mater 1993;9(4):274–9.

[23] Taskonak B, Mecholsky JJ Jr, Anusavice KJ. Residual stresses in bilayer dental ceramics. Biomaterials 2005;26(16):3235–41.

[24] Kelly JR. Clinically relevant approach to failure testing of all-ceramic restorations. J Prosthet Dent 1999;8(6):652–61.

[25] Zhang Y, Song JK, Lawn BR. Deep-penetrating conical cracks in brittle layers from hydraulic cyclic contact. J Biomed Mater Res B Appl Biomater 2005;73(1):186–93.

[26] Kelly JR, Campbell SD, Bowen HK. Fracture-surface analysis of dental ceramics. J Prosthet Dent 1989;62(5):536–41.

[27] Quinn JB, Quinn GD, Kelly JR, et al. Fractographic analyses of three ceramic whole crown restoration failures. Dent Mater 2005;21(10):920–9.

[28] Thompson JY, Anusavice KJ, Naman A, et al. Fracture surface characterization of clinically failed all-ceramic crowns. J Dent Res 1994;73(12):1824–32.

[29] Scherrer SS, Quinn JB, Quinn GD, et al. Failure analysis of ceramic clinical cases using qualitative fractography. Int J Prosthodont 2006;19(2):185–92.

[30] Scherrer SS, Quinn JB, Quinn GD, et al. Fractographic ceramic failure analysis using the replica technique. Dent Mater 2007, in press.

[31] Flanders LA, Quinn JB, Wilson OC Jr, et al. Scratch hardness and chipping of dental ceramics under different environments. Dent Mater 2003;19(8):716–24.

[32] Qasim T, Ford C, Bush MB, et al. Margin failures in brittle dome structures: relevance to failure of dental crowns. J Biomed Mater Res B Appl Biomater in press, published online August 29, 2005.

[33] ASTM. C1239-06a standard practice for reporting uniaxial strength data and estimating Weibull distribution parameters for advanced ceramics. Annual book of ASTM standards. Philadelphia: American Society for Testing Materials; 2006. p. 309–15.

[34] Thoman DR, Bain LJ, Antle CE. Inferences on the parameters of the Weibull distribution. Technometrics 1969;11:445–60.

[35] Kaplan EL, Meier P. Nonparametric estimation from incomplete observations. J Am Stat Assoc 1958;53:457–81.

[36] Barnes D, Gingell JC, George D, et al. Clinical evaluation of an all-ceramic restorative system: 24-month report. Am J Dent 2006;19(4):206–10.

[37] Bindl A, Mormann WH. Survival rate of mono-ceramic and ceramic-core CAD/CAM-generated anterior crowns over 2–5 years. Eur J Oral Sci 2004;112(2):197–204.

[38] Bindl A, Richter B, Mormann WH. Survival of ceramic computer-aided design/manufacturing crowns bonded to preparations with reduced macroretention geometry. Int J Prosthodont 2005;18(3):219–24.

[39] Coelho Santos MJ, Mondelli RF, Lauris JR, et al. Clinical evaluation of ceramic inlays and onlays fabricated with two systems: two-year clinical follow up. Oper Dent 2004;29(2):123–30.

[40] Esquivel-Upshaw JF, Anusavice KJ, Young H, et al. Clinical performance of a lithia disilicate-based core ceramic for three-unit posterior FPDs. Int J Prosthodont 2004;17(4):469–75.

[41] Fradeani M, Redemagni M, Corrado M. Porcelain laminate veneers: 6- to 12-year clinical evaluation—a retrospective study. Int J Periodontics Restorative Dent 2005;25(1):9–17.

[42] Kaytan B, Onal B, Pamir T, et al. Clinical evaluation of indirect resin composite and ceramic onlays over a 24-month period. Gen Dent 2005;53(5):329–34.

[43] Krämer N, Ebert J, Petschelt A, et al. Ceramic inlays bonded with two adhesive after 4 years. Dent Mater 2006;22(1):13–21.

[44] Krämer N, Frankenberger R. Clinical performance of bonded leucite-reinforced glass ceramic inlays and onlays after eight years. Dent Mater 2005;21(3):262–71.

[45] Marquardt P, Strub JR. Survival rates of IPS empress 2 all-ceramic crowns and fixed partial dentures: results of a 5-year prospective clinical study. Quintessence Int 2006;37(4):253–9.

[46] Schulte AG, Vockler A, Reinhardt R. Longevity of ceramic inlays and onlays luted with a solely light-curing composite resin. J Dent 2005;33(5):433–42.

[47] Sjogren G, Molin M, van Dijken JW. A 10-year prospective evaluation of CAD/CAM-manufactured (Cerec) ceramic inlays cemented with a chemically cured or dual-cured resin composite. Int J Prosthodont 2004;17(2):241–6.

[48] Smales RJ, Etemadi S. Long-term survival of porcelain laminate veneers using two preparation designs: a retrospective study. Int J Prosthodont 2004;17(3):323–6.

[49] Suarez MJ, Lozano JF, Paz Salido M, et al. Three-year clinical evaluation of In-Ceram Zirconia posterior FPDs. Int J Prosthodont 2004;17(1):35–8.

[50] Taskonak B, Sertgoz A. Two-year clinical evaluation of lithia-disilicate-based all-ceramic crowns and fixed partial dentures. Dent Mater in press, published online December 19, 2005.

[51] Thordrup M, Isidor F, Horsted-Bindslev P. A prospective clinical study of indirect and direct composite and ceramic inlays: ten-year results. Quintessence Int 2006;37(2):139–44.

[52] Vult von Steyern P, Carlson P, Nilner K. All-ceramic fixed partial dentures designed according to the DC-Zirkon technique. A 2-year clinical study. J Oral Rehabil 2005;32(3):180–7.

[53] Walter MH, Wolf BH, Wolf AE, et al. Six-year clinical performance of all-ceramic crowns with alumina cores. Int J Prosthodont 2006;19(2):162–3.

[54] Wolfart S, Bohlsen F, Wegner SM, et al. A preliminary prospective evaluation of all-ceramic crown-retained and inlay-retained fixed partial dentures. Int J Prosthodont 2005;18(6): 497–505.

[55] Zarone F, Sorrentino R, Vaccaro F, et al. Retrospective clinical evaluation of 86 Procera AllCeram anterior single crowns on natural and implant-supported abutments. Clin Implant Dent Relat Res 2005;7(Suppl 1):S95–103.

[56] Reich SM, Wichmann M, Rinne H, et al. Clinical performance of large, all-ceramic CAD/CAM-generated restorations after three years: a pilot study. J Am Dent Assoc 2004; 135(5):605–12.

[57] Hayashi M, Tsubakimoto Y, Takeshige F, et al. Analysis of longitudinal marginal deterioration of ceramic inlays. Oper Dent 2004;29(4):386–91.

ELSEVIER
SAUNDERS

THE DENTAL
CLINICS
OF NORTH AMERICA

Dent Clin N Am 51 (2007) 729–746

Bone Graft Materials

Harry V. Precheur, DMD[a,b,*]

[a]Department of Oral and Maxillofacial Surgery and Pathology, University of Mississippi
Medical Center, 2500 North State Street, Jackson, MS 39216-4505, USA
[b]Department of Surgery, Division of Plastic and Reconstructive Surgery, University of
Mississippi Medical Center, 2500 North State Street, Jackson, MS 39216-4505, USA

The replacement of bone is a complex and demanding undertaking. A brief description of bone's biology and constitutional elements is helpful in understanding the challenges that must be met when its replacement by grafting is the goal. Bone formation occurs when osteoblasts secrete collagen molecules and ground substance. The collagen molecules polymerize to form collagen fibers. Calcium salts precipitate in the ground substance along the collagen fibers to form osteoid. Osteoblasts become trapped in the osteoid and then are called osteocytes.

Mature compact bone is composed of approximately 30% organic matrix and 70% calcium salts. Ninety percent to 95% of the organic matrix is collagen fibers, and the remainder is the gelatinous medium called ground substance, which is composed of chondroitin sulfate and hyaluronic acid. The collagen fibers are oriented along the lines of tensional force. The predominant crystalline salt, composed of calcium and phosphate, is hydroxyapatite—$CA10 (P04)6 (OH) 2$. Compact bone has hydroxyapatite crystals lying adjacent to and bound to the collagen fibers. The collagen fibers provide tensile strength, and the hydroxyapatite crystals provide compressional strength [1]. Duplication of these constitutional elements comprises some of the grafting materials discussed later in this article.

Bone formation in grafting is characterized by three types of bone growth: osteogenesis, osteoinduction, and osteoconduction. Osteogenesis is the formation of new bone by osteoblasts derived from the graft material itself. Osteoinduction is the ability of a material to induce the formation of osteoblasts from the surrounding tissue at the graft host site, which results in

---

* Department of Oral and Maxillofacial Surgery and Pathology, University of Mississippi
Medical Center, 2500 North State Street, Jackson, MS 39216-4505.
E-mail address: hprecheur@sod.umsmed.edu

0011-8532/07/$ - see front matter © 2007 Elsevier Inc. All rights reserved.
doi:10.1016/j.cden.2007.03.004
dental.theclinics.com

bone growth. Osteoconduction is the ability of a material to support the growth of bone over a surface.

Although not directly responsible for bone formation, an additional characteristic, osteointegration, which is the ability to chemically bind to the surrounding bone, is desirable to aid in the incorporation of the graft at the host site.

Autogenous bone grafts

Autogenous bone grafts, also called autografts, are bone grafts transferred from one site to another site within the same individual. These grafts are the gold standard to which all other grafting materials are compared because they possess all of the previously mentioned characteristics. Because they are from the host itself, there is also an absence of antigenicity.

Autogenous grafts can be cortical or cancellous or a combination of both. Cancellous grafts have the ability to revascularize sooner because of their spongy architecture. This revascularization begins at around the fifth day [2]. Before revascularization, cellular survival in the graft depends on nutrition and elimination of metabolic waste products through plasmatic diffusion. Osteocytes within their lacunae seem to survive if they are within 0.3 mm of a perfusion surface [3]. Cortical grafts require considerable resorption by osteoclastic activity before osteoblastic bone formation. This process is called "creeping substitution" and can produce areas of necrotic bone that persist indefinitely [4].

As a result of the differing biology of cortical and cancellous bone, the characteristics of a graft composed of each type differ. A cortical graft is strong initially but weakens overtime before regaining strength. There also may be a loss of dimension as a result of a resorption process unless physiologic stress stimulation is producing bone reorganization. Dynamic loading has been shown to be critical for the preservation and increase of bone mass in vivo and, on a cellular level, for modulation of osteoblastic and osteoclastic activity [5,6]. Cortical grafts have been shown to be 40% to 50% weaker than normal bone from 6 weeks to 6 months after transplantation [2]. Cancellous grafts tend to be weak initially because of their open architecture but continually gain in strength. Physiologic stress stimulation is necessary for continued dimensional and strength stability.

The disadvantages of autogenous grafts are the amount of available graft material and the morbidity associated with their harvest. These disadvantages have led to the development of myriad grafting materials that can be classified into the following categories:

Allografts, also called allogenic, homologous, or homografts, are composed of materials taken from another individual of the same species.
Xenografts, also known as heterografts or xenogenic grafts, are materials taken from another species.

Alloplastic grafts, or synthetic grafts, are artificial or manufactured materials and can be subdivided based on their origin and chemical composition.

There are many and varied combinations of these materials (see list). This article examines each class of material based on some of the studies in each of the following categories: safety, animal research, periodontal and maxillofacial applications, skeletal grafting, and attempt to qualify the efficacy of each class of material. The article also examines some of the research being done in "tissue engineering" to get a sense of the future of bone grafting.

Allografts

Allografts are cadaveric in origin. This type of grafting material is attractive because it closely matches the recipient in constitutional elements and architecture and is theoretically available in unlimited quality. The fundamental problems of this grafting material are antigenicity and the potential for transmission of disease.

Although allografts are treated in various ways, the real and perceived risk of disease transmission still exists. It has been estimated that the risk of HIV transmission is 1 in 1.6 million [7]. There has been one reported case of hepatitis B and three cases of hepatitis C transmission associated with the transplantation of allografts, with the latest case occurring in 1992 [8]. There have been two separate cases of septic arthritis from bone-tendon-bone allografts from a common donor for reconstruction of anterior cruciate ligaments [9]. The US Centers for Disease Control and Prevention conducted an investigation that revealed at least 25 other cases of allograft-related infection or illness [10].

As recently as March 9, 2006, there was a recall of allograft regenerative products produced by manufacturers, including Tutogen Inc., Regeneration Technologies Inc., Lifecell Corp., Lost Mountain Tissue Bank, and the Blood and Tissue Center of Central Texas. This recall resulted from an investigation of Biomedical Tissue Services, Ltd., a New Jersey company under scrutiny for allegedly procuring tissue from funeral homes without proper documentation [11]. Recalled tissues were tested for HIV, hepatitis B virus, and hepatitis C virus, and as of March 2006, no contaminated allografts were identified [12]. Despite these risks and in recognition of the advantages of bone grafting using allograft material, bone grafting procedures expanded from approximately 10,000 cases in 1985 to more than 1 million in 2004 [5,13].

Allografts for maxillofacial and periodontal use generally come as demineralized freeze-dried bone allografts (DFDBA) or mineralized freeze-dried bone allografts (FDBA) and in the form of particles, sheets, blocks, or entire preformed bones. Some researchers propose that removal of the mineral component allows greater expression of osteoinductive proteins [13–16]; however, allografts are predominately space-occupying osteoconductive lattices or frameworks. The osteoinductive capability of these products is minimal because of the low concentration of bone growth proteins as a result of the rigorous processes involved in the removal of potential antigenicity and pathogenicity [17]. Piatell and colleagues [18] found that only the DFDBA particles near the host bone were involved in the mineralization process, whereas in FDBA even particles that were farthest from the host bone were lined by osteoblasts actively secreting osteoid matrix and newly formed bone. No osteoinduction was observed with FDBA or DFDBA. There was an increased osteoconductive effect with FDBA.

Noumbissi and colleagues [19] compared mineralized cancellous allograft material to a 1:1 combination of DFDBA and deproteinized mineralized bovine bone in bilateral sinus grafts and concluded that resorption and replacement by new bone occurred more rapidly in the mineralized cancellous allograft material but that both groups resulted in successful new bone formation. Two years after completion of the study there were no differences in osteointegration or stability of implants placed in either material. Schwartz and colleagues [20] demonstrated that different bone bank preparation of DFDBA, even from the same bank, varied considerably in their ability to induce new bone formation and further concluded that the ability to induce bone formation seems to depend on the donor age. Fucini and colleagues [21] studied allograft particle size and found no statistically significant difference in bone fill in periodontal osseous defects between different particle sizes of DFBA in humans. Glowacki [22] stated that we cannot conclude what the performance of different lots of demineralized bone allografts will be in vivo or in vitro and that test systems should be used as a measure of clinical performance. The author also called for an osteoconductivity standard for products that are to be released to market followed by clinical monitoring.

Animal studies have demonstrated (1) improved skeletal healing in mice with the use of demineralized bone matrix + hyaluronan [23], (2) better bone fill in critical-sized defects in baboons using DFDBA combined with tendonous collagen [24], (3) stable augmentation of the sinus floor with the use of deproteinized bone particles in rabbits [25], (4) comparable mechanical loading of implants with the use of homogeneous demineralized freeze-dried bone in one-stage sinus lift procedures in sheep when compared with autogenous cancellous bone from the iliac crest [26], and (5) new bone formation induced by active DFDBA and a dose-dependent increase in new bone area that exceeded that induced by active DFDBA caused by the addition of rhBMP-2 to inactive DFDBA [27].

Human studies and case reports of the use of these materials in the maxillofacial region have yielded the following information:

Ridge augmentation and sinus grafting with freeze-dried bone allograft in combination with platelet-rich plasma provides a therapeutic alternative for implant placement [28].

Mineralized, solvent dehydrated cancellous bone allografts were replaced by newly formed bone significantly faster and in greater quantities in the maxillary sinus when compared with a composite of DFDBA plus deproteinized bovine bone xenografts [19].

Allogenic bone block material is an effective alternative to autogenous bone for implant site development [29].

Van Den Bergh and colleagues [30] reported the placement of 69 implants in 30 sinuses grafted with DFDB without the loss of a single implant.

Minichetti and colleagues [31] studied the grafting of extraction sockets with particulate mineralized bone allograft and concluded that it demonstrated the formation or remodeling of bone and was clinically useful in maintaining bone volume for implant placement after extraction.

Grogan and colleagues [32] reported that "allograft bone produced reliable results with a satisfactory outcome" in posterior spinal fusion for correction of idiopathic scoliosis.

Cammisa and colleagues [33] compared a demineralized bone gel to iliac crest autogenous grafts, with each patient acting as his or her own control. They found bone fusion in 52% of the allograft side and 54% of the autogenous side.

Summary

Although the results of these studies do not yield consistent results, they demonstrate that allografts are osteoconductive and some are possibly osteoinductive. Under the right circumstances and with proper patient and site selection, they provide an acceptable material for grafting.

Xenografts

The disadvantages of allografts, including disease transmission, antigenicity, supply, and psychological aversion, have led to the exploration of xenografts as an alternative grafting material. Xenografts are bovine in origin and carry the theoretical risk of transmission of bovine spongiform encephalopathy. Theoretical and experimental data, however, indicate that the use of these materials does not carry a risk for transmitting bovine spongiform encephalopathy to humans [34]. Sogal and Tofe [35] applied the risk assessment models of the German Federal Ministry of Health and the Pharmaceutical Research and Manufacturers Association of America to a bovine bone graft substitute and concluded that the risk of bovine spongiform encephalopathy transmission was negligible. This was attributed to the stringent protocols followed in sourcing and processing.

Animal studies have revealed the following information:

Bovine bone granules possess better osteoconductive potential than bioglass crystals and hydroxyapatite when tested in New Zealand rabbits [36].

Xenogenic demineralized bone matrix was osteoconductive when implanted in rats [37].

Bovine bone xenograft was to be more effective than particulate dentin combined with plaster of Paris in forming new bone in calvarial bone defects in rats [38].

Xenographic grafts undergo slower resorption than autogenous grafts when placed in mandibular lateral surface defects in dogs [39].

Xenografts were essentially osteoconductive when examined in monkeys [40].

Human use of xenografts has demonstrated the following findings:

Bovine bone mineral grafts, when used with barrier membranes, improved clinical and radiographic parameters of deep intrabony pockets [41].

Excellent integration of inorganic bovine material with newly formed bone suggests that the material can be used for onlay grafting procedures [42].

Biocompatibility and successful use occur in rebuilding atrophic alveolar ridges when supported by a configured titanium mesh [43].

Success in sinus elevation procedures with or without implant placement occurs when used alone or in combination with venous blood, platelet rich plasma, and autogenous bone [44–54].

A unique regenerative product combines an anorganic bovine bone matrix with Pepgen-15 (P-15), a synthetic peptide that mimics the cell-binding domain of type 1 collagen [55,56]. Because collagen forms the scaffold for cell attachment—migration—and modulates cell differentiation and morphogenesis by mediating the flux of chemical and mechanical stimuli and because the P-15 peptide represents the cell-binding site of collagen, it was hypothesized that materials coated with P-15 should act as an effective substitute for autogenous bone grafts [57]. Bhatnagar and colleagues [56] have demonstrated that this material produced enhanced bone formation within a shorter time interval compared with a composite graft material composed of anorganic bovine bone and DFDBA. Thompson and colleagues [58] compared a P-15 product to mineralized FDBA and coralline hydroxyapatite in 13 maxillary extraction sockets and found that the P-15–containing grafts produced the highest amount of vital bone. Human osteoblasts have been shown to demonstrate the greatest proliferation and differentiation in vitro when applied to a P-15–containing graft material as compared with coralline hydroxyapatite, low temperature bovine hydroxyapatite, alpha tricalcium phosphate, and high-temperature bovine hydroxyapatite [59,60]. Similar results were demonstrated when P-15 was combined with hydroxyapatite calcified from red algae [61].

Alloplasts

Alloplastic materials that have been investigated and manufactured include hydroxyapatite, coral- and algae-derived hydroxyapatite, the calcium phosphates, calcium sulfate, collagen, and polymers. These synthetic materials are inert with no or little osteoinductive activity, with the exception of P-15, which is claimed to stimulate the differentiation of mesenchymal cells into osteoblasts [59–61].

The advantages of alloplastic grafts include an absence of antigenicity, no potential for disease transmission, and unlimited supply. These materials can be treated to be resorbable or nonresorbable, are provided in various particle or pore sizes, are combined with various carriers to improve handling characteristics, or are combined with bioactive proteins to provide osteoinduction. Animal studies of these materials have demonstrated the following findings:

Bone formation in monkey extraction sites and dog infrabony periodontal defects with a hydroxyapatite/agarose gel [62,63].

Bone fill in rat calvarial defects, when hydroxyapatite was combined with chitosan glutamate [64], cultured bone marrow osteoblasts [65], and reconstituted collagen microspheres [66].

Mineralization rates for nanoparticle hydroxyapatite that were comparable to autogenous bone in pig osseous defects [67].

Bone formation with porous hydroxyapatite in posterolateral lumbar fusion in sheep [68].

Human studies revealed these findings:

Hydroxyapatite bone cement seems to hold great promise as a grafting alloplastic material for sinus floor augmentations [69].

Hydroxyapatite can be used as a porous ceramic or as a paste/cement bone graft material in humans in the hand [70], cranium [71], and tibia [72,73].

Coral- and algae-derived hydroxyapatite

Because coral- and algae-derived hydroxyapatite has similar architecture and similar mechanical properties to cancellous bone, much research has gone into its use as a substitute graft material on its own or combined with other substances [74]. Unlike bone, coral's inorganic component is calcium carbonate, which can be exchanged for phosphate to produce coralline hydroxyapatite [75]. Like other synthetic materials, coral- and algae-derived hydroxyapatite is not osteoinductive or osteogenic [76]. Its structure and composition mimic natural bone, however [74]. Pore size and interconnectivity and particle size have been shown to influence bone regeneration and growth [77]. A minimum pore size of 100 nm is required for ingrowth of connective tissue or osteoid, with an ideal pore size of approximately 100 to 135 nm [78,79].

The rate of a material's resorption is a critical element in a graft's success as the material maintains a desired volume that should be replaced with bone. Premature resorption of graft material may result in inadequate volume of the replacement [80,81]. This rate of resorption is influenced by porosity and the composition of the graft material [82–84].

Simunek and colleagues [85] demonstrated that a material derived from sea algae was gradually resorbed and replaced by newly formed bone. Ewers and colleagues showed that marine-derived hydroxyapatite material combined with 10% autogenous bone and plasma-rich protein produced comparable—and in some cases better—results than autogenous grafts in sinus augmentation procedures [81]. Similar results were obtained with the use of this material in the foot and ankle [86] and iliac crest [87]. Less promising results were produced when it was used for spinal fusion in rabbits [88] and humans [89].

Bioactive glass

Bioactive glasses were introduced more than 30 years ago as bone substitutes. The designation "bioactive" relates to their ability to bond to bone and enhance bone-tissue formation. This is thought to be a result of the similarity of surface composition and structure of the bioactive materials to the mineral component of bone. This bioactivity depends on an intimate contact with bone and is limited in nature [90]. Because of these characteristics, studies have used this material as stand-alone bone grafting materials and scaffolds for osteoinductive proteins and osteogenic cells. The rate and degree of resorption are a function of architecture, particle size, and manufacturing methods [83].

Research in animals has yielded conflicting results.

Moreira-Gonzalez and colleagues [91] concluded that "the use of bioglass granules to repair large craniofacial defects cannot be advised." This statement was based the study of the repair of critical sized calvarial defects in rabbits.

Griffin and colleagues [92] looked at metaphyseal defects in sheep and found that defects filled with mixtures that contained 50% to 100% bioactive glass contained less bone and more fibrous tissue than defects filled with allograft, autograft, or allograft combined (<50%) with bioglass.

Hall and colleagues [93] found no statistically significant difference between bioactive glass and no material in the repair of intrabony defects around implants in the canine mandible and found that DFDBA produced better bone to implant contact and better bone height fill than bioactive glass material.

Other studies have come to different conclusions:

Wheeler and colleagues [94] studied critical sized distal femoral cancellous bone defects treated with bioactive glasses and found that all grafted defects had more bone than unfilled controls.

Cancian and colleagues [95] found total repair of surgically created defects in monkey mandibles with intimate contact of the remaining particles of bioactive glass and newly formed bone at 180 days.

Research on the use of bioactive glass in spinal fusion in rabbits has led others to conclude that it may have potential as a bone graft material [96,97].

When this material was looked at for improved healing in extraction sockets or sinus floor augmentation, either alone or in combination with other grafting materials (DFDBA, autogenous bone), it was found to be effective for bone regeneration [98–104].

Calcium phosphates and calcium sulfate

Calcium phosphate is the name given to a group of minerals that contain calcium ions (Ca 2+) combined with orthophosphates (PO4 3−). Tricalcium phosphate Ca3 (PO4)2, which is also known as Whitlockite, occurs in alpha and beta phases [105]. Hydroxyapatite, Ca10 (PO4) [6], (OH)2 is the principle mineral component of bone [1]. Calcium sulfate (CaS04) is better known as plaster of Paris or gypsum and has been used as synthetic bone graft material for more than 100 years [106].

Calcium sulfate

Human studies most recently have concentrated on the use of this material in combination with other graft materials. Maragos and colleagues [107] looked at its use combined with doxycycline and DFDBA in the treatment of class II mandibular furcation defects in humans and found that either of these additions significantly enhanced the clinical outcome than did calcium sulfate alone. Borrelli and colleagues [108] concluded that medical grade calcium sulfate increases the volume of graft material, facilitates bone formation, and is safe in the treatment of nonunions and fractures with osseous defects. Other researchers also have demonstrated this material's biocompatibility and osteoconduction [109,110]. Herron and colleagues [111] demonstrated resorption of calcium phosphate and its replacement with bone in rabbits.

Calcium phosphate

Blokhuis and colleagues [112] compared calcium phosphate with autogenous bone grafts in 3-cm tibial segmental defects in sheep and concluded that calcium phosphate does not provide an alternative to autogenous grafts for this use. Linhart and colleagues [113] concluded that calcium phosphate cements represent a good alternative to autogenous bone transplantation, especially in elderly patients.

Tricalcium phosphate has been shown to have no adverse effect on cell count, viability, and morphology and can provide a matrix that favors limited cell proliferation in vitro [114]. Rabbit 1-cm diaphyseal segmental defects treated with calcium sulfate combined with mesenchymal stem cells gave evidence of the use of this material as an alternative to autografts [115]. When tricalcium phosphate was compared with inorganic bovine bone in dog mandibular defects, tricalcium phosphate showed significantly greater bone formation at 12 and 24 months and better resorption than inorganic bovine bone [116]. Several studies in human sinus augmentation, either alone or in combination with other substances, have demonstrated its use as an effective bone grafting material [117–122]. Ultraporus beta tricalcium phosphate used in 24 patients with orthopedic bone cavity defects exhibited steady resorption and trabeculation with time, but incorporation was not complete at 1 year in large defects [123].

The future

Current avenues of research in molecular biology, progenitor cell use, and biomimetic scaffolds hold promise for the future of bone replacements by defining and employing the complex of stimuli and processes that can result in bone formation. Postnatal progenitor cells have demonstrated the capacity to differentiate into a multitude of cell types [124–126]. Mesenchymal stem cells can be harvested from bone marrow and demonstrate extensive proliferative ability and the capacity to be guided into bone-forming cell types [124]. Their availability is a limiting factor because their fraction in marrow has been estimated to be as low as 1 in 27,000 cells [127,128]. Adipose tissue–derived progenitor cells also have been investigated [129–131]. They possess the advantages of availability and accessibility and have demonstrated capabilities similar to bone marrow–derived cells. In vitro and in vivo studies have demonstrated their ability to form bone [130–132].

The molecular processes of the multitude of factors in platelet rich plasma, pro-osteogenic cytokines (BMP 2, 4, 7), and angiogenic factors leading to osteoblastic bone formation are being elucidated [133,134]. The delivery or support of these biochemicals or cellular elements depends on a carrier or scaffolding system. Collagen, hyaluronic acid, calcium phosphate, chitosan, and hydroxyapatite have been studied in the past [135–138]. Polymer chemistry has yielded polyglycolic acid, polylactic acid, polycaplactone, and combinations such as the copolymer polyglycolic acid–polylactic acid. Although these polymers are biocompatible, their breakdown products are potentially tissue damaging.

The goal is to configure these materials as competent carriers of the biomolecular pro-osteogenics or as supportive scaffolds for cellular proliferation and bone formation [139–142]. One technique that is showing some promise is three-dimensional printing technology. Three-dimensional complex shapes or structures can be computer generated, constructed in a three-dimensional printer, and then used as protein or cellular carriers for custom implantable bone graft substitutes.

Summary

A plethora of products on the market is designed to be used for the replacement or grafting of human bone. Each clinician must select the best product for its particular advantages when used for a defined purpose in patients. Careful review of the research underpinnings for each product is essential when considering its use. Because the substance that is the equivalent of the autogenous bone graft has yet to be developed, continued research of materials and material combinations is helping us understand the complex of interconnected elements that are essential for successful grafting. As our understanding of these processes matures, there is great hope for the development of the "ideal" substitute for the autogenous bone graft.

References

[1] Guyton AG, Hall JE. Textbook of medical physiology. Philadelphia: W.B. Saunders; 2000. p. 901–4.

[2] Wilk RM. Bony reconstruction of the jaws. In: Miloro M, editor. Peterson's principles of oral and maxillofacial surgery. 2nd edition. Hamilton (London): B C Decker; 2004. p. 785–7.

[3] Heslop BK, Zeiss IM, Nisbet NW. Studies on transference of bone: a comparison of autologous and homologous transplants with reference to osteocyte survival osteogenesis and host reaction. Br J Exp Pathol 1960;41:269–72.

[4] Enneking WF, Burcharot H, Puhl JJ, et al. Physical and biological aspects of repair in dog cortical-bone transplants. J Bone Joint Surg 1975;57:237–52.

[5] Oxlund H, Anderson NB, Ortoft G, et al. Growth hormone and mild exercise in combination markedly enhances cortical bone formation and strength in old rats. Endocrinology 1998;139(4):1899–904.

[6] Duncan RL, Turner CH. Mechanotransduction and the functional of bone to mechanical strain. Calcif Tissue Int 1995;57(5):344–58.

[7] Boyce T, Edwards J, Scarborough N. Allograft bone: the influence of processing on safety and performance. Orthop Clin North Am 1999;30(4):571–81.

[8] Tomford WW. Transmission of disease through transplantation of musculoskeletal allografts. J Bone Joint Surg Am 1995;77–A(11):1742j–54j.

[9] CDC First Document, Center for Disease Control. Septic arthritis following anterior cruciate ligament reconstruction using tendon allografts, Florida and Louisiana 2000. Morb Mortal Wkly Rep 2001;50(48):1081–3.

[10] CDC Second Document, Center for Disease Control. Update: allograft associated bacterial infections: United States, 2002. Morb Mortal Wkly Rep 2002;51(10):207–10.

[11] National Tissue Product Recall Impact Continues For OMS, Patients. AAOMS Today January–February 2006:3.

[12] E-mail AAOMS March 2006.

[13] Bolander ME, Balian G. The use of demineralized bone matrix in the repair of segmental defects: augmentation with extracted matrix proteins and a comparison with autologous grafts. J Bone Joint Surg 1986;68–A:1264–74.

[14] Hopp SG, Dahners LE, Gilbert JA. A study of mechanical strength of long bone defects treated with various bone autograft substitutes: an experimental investigation in the rabbit. J Orthop Res 1989;7(4):578–84.

[15] Urist MR, Chang JJ, Leitze A, et al. Preparation and bioassay of bone morphogenic protein and polypetides fragments. Methods Enzymol 1987;146:294–312.

[16] Russel JL. Allografts and osteoinductivity. Presented at the European Federation of National Associations of Orthopaedics and Traumatology, Technical Symposium on "Demineralized Bone Allografts and Osteoinduction". Rhodes, June 4, 2001.

[17] Wozney JM. Bone morphogenic proteins and their gene expression. In: Masaki N, editor. Cellular and molecular biology of bone. Tokyo: Academic Press, Inc; 1993. p. 131–67.

[18] Piattelli A, Scarano M, Corigliano M, et al. Comparison of bone regeneration with the use of mineralized and demineralized freeze-dried bone allografts: a histological and histo-chemical study in man. In: Masaki N, editor. Biomaterials 1996;17(14):1127–31.

[19] Noumbissi SS, Lozada JL, Boyne PJ, et al. Clinical histologic and histomorphometric evaluation of mineralized solvent-dehydrated bone allograft in human maxillary sinus grafts. J Oral Implantol 2005;31(4):171–9.

[20] Schwartz Z, Somers A, Mellonig JT, et al. Ability of commercial demineralized freeze-dried bone allograft to induce new bone formation is dependent on donor age but not gender. J Periodontol 1998;69(4):470–8.

[21] Fucini SE, Quintero G, Gher ME, et al. Small versus large particles of demineralized freeze-dried bone allografts in human intrabony periodontal defects. J Periodontol 1993;64(9):844–7.

[22] Glowacki J. A review of osteoinductive testing methods and sterilization processes for demineralized bone. Cell Tissue Bank 2005;6(1):3–12.

[23] Colnot C, Romero DM, Huang S, et al. Mechanisms of action of demineralized bone matrix in the repair of cortical bone defects. Clin Orthop Relat Res 2005;(435):69–78.

[24] Kohles SS, Vernino AR, Clagett JA, et al. A morphometric evaluation of allograft matrix combinations in the treatment of osseous defects in a baboon model. Calcif Tissue Int 2000; 67(2):156–62.

[25] XU H, Shimizu Y, Asal S, et al. Grafting of deproteinized bone particles inhibits bone resorption after maxillary sinus elevation. Clin Oral Implants Res 2004;15(1):126–33.

[26] Haas R, Haidvogl D, Dortbudak O, et al. Freeze dried bone for maxillary sinus augmentation in sheep. Clin Oral Implants Res 2002;13(6):581–6.

[27] Schwartz Z, Somers A, Mellonig JT, et al. Addition of human recombinant bone morphogenic protein-2 to inactive commercial human demineralized freeze-dried bone allograft makes an effective composite bone inductive implant material. J Periodontol 1998;69(12):1337–45.

[28] Kassolis JD, Rosen PS, Reynolds MA. Alveolar ridge and sinus augmentation utilizing platelet-rich plasma in combination with freeze-dried bone allograft: case series. J Periodontal 2000;71(10):1654–61.

[29] Leonetti JA, Koup R. Localized maxillary ridge augmentation with a block allograft for dental implant placement: case reports. Implant Dent 2003;12(3):217–26.

[30] Van Den Berch JP, Ten Bruggenkate CM, Krekeler G, et al. Maxillary sinus floor elevation and grafting with human demineralized freeze-dried bone. Clin Oral Implants Res 2000; 11(5):487–93.

[31] Minichetti JC, D'Amore JC, Honga YJ, et al. Human histologic analysis of mineralized bone allograft placement before implant surgery. J Oral Implantol 2004;30(2):74–82.

[32] Grogan DP, Kalen V, Ross TL, et al. Use of allograft bone for posterior spinal fusion in idiopathic scoliosis. Clin Orthop Relat Res 1999;(369):273–8.

[33] Cammisa FP Jr, Lowery G, Garfin SR, et al. Two year fusion rate equivalency between grafton DBM gel and autograft in posterior lateral spine fusion: a prospective controlled trial employing a side by side comparison in the same patient. Spine 2004;29(6):660–6.

[34] Wenz B, Oesch B, Horst M. Analysis of the risk of transmitting bovine spongiform encephalopathy through bone grafts derived from bovine bone. Biomaterials 2001;22(12):1599–606.

[35] Sogal A, Tofe AJ. Risk assessment of bovine spongiform encephalopathy transmission through bone graft material derived from bovine bone used for dental applications. J Periodontol 1999;70(9):1053–63.

[36] Al Ruhaimi KA. Bone graft substitutes: a comparative qualitative histologic review of current osteoconductive grafting materials. Int J Oral Maxillofac Implants 2001;16(1):105–14.

[37] Torricelli P, Fini M, Rocca M, et al. Xenogenic demineralized bone matrix: osteoinduction an influence of associated skeletal defects in heterotopic bone formation in rats. Int Orthop 1999;23(3):178–81.

[38] Su-Gwan K, Hak-Kyun K, Sung-Chul L. Combined implantation of particulate dentine, plaster of Paris, and a bone xenograft (Bio-Oss) for bone regeneration in rats. J Craniomaxillofac Surg 2001;29(5):282–8.

[39] Araujo MG, Sonohara M, Hayacibara R, et al. Lateral ridge augmentation by the use of grafts comprised of autologous bone or a biomaterial: an experiment in the dog. J Clin Periodontol 2002;29(12):1122–31.

[40] Hammerle CH, Chiantella GC, Karring T, et al. The effect of a deproteinized bovine bone mineral on bone regeneration around titanium dental implants. Clin Oral Implants Res 1998;9(3):151–62.

[41] Vouros I, Aristodimou E, Konstantinidis A. Guided tissue regeneration in intrabony periodontal defects following treatment with two bioabsorbable membranes in combination with bovine bone mineral graft: a clinical and radiographic study. J Clin Perodontal 2004;31(10):908–17.

[42] Proussaefs P, Lozada J, Rohrer MD. A clinical and histologic evaluation of a block onlay graft in conjunction with autogenous particulate and inorganic bovine material (Bio-Oss): a case report. Int J Periodontics Restorative Dent 2002;22(6):567–73.

[43] Artzi Z, Dayan D, Alpern Y, et al. Vertical ridge augmentation using xenogenic material supported by a configured titanium mesh: clinicohistopathologic and histochemical study. Int J Oral Maxillofac Implants 2003;18(3):4440–6.

[44] Yildirim M, Spiekermann H, Handt S, et al. Maxillary sinus augmentation with the xenograft Bio-Oss and autogenous intraoral bone for qualitative improvement of the implant site: a histologic and histomorphometric clinical study in humans. Int J Oral Maxillofac Implants 2001;16(1):23–33.

[45] Valentini P, Abensur D, Wenz B, et al. Sinus grafting with porous bone mineral (Bio-Oss) for implant placement: a 5-year study on 15 patients. Int J Periodontics Restorative Dent 2000;20(3):245–53.

[46] Yildirim M, Spiekermann H, Biesterfeld S, et al. Maxillary sinus augmentation using xenogenic bone substitute material Bio-OSS in combination with venous blood: a histologic and histomorphometric study in humans. Clin Oral Implants Res 2000;11(3):217–29.

[47] Hallman M, Cederlund A, Lindskog S, et al. A clinical histologic study of bovine hydroxyapatite in combination with autogenous bone and fibrin glue for maxillary sinus floor augmentation: results after 6 to 8 months of healing. Clin Oral Implants Res 2001;12(2):135–43.

[48] Sanchez AR, Eckert SE, Sheridan PJ, et al. Influence of platelet-rich plasma added to xenogeneic bone grafts on bone mineral density associated with dental implants. Int J Oral Maxillofac Implants 2005;20(4):526–32.

[49] Tadjoedin ES, De Lange GL, Bronckers AL, et al. Deproteinized cancellous bovine bone (Bio-Oss) as bone substitute for sinus floor elevation: a retrospective, histomorphometrical study of five cases. J Clin Periodontol 2003;30(3):261–70.

[50] Kasabah S, Simunek A, Krug J, et al. Maxillary sinus augmentation with deproteinized bovine bone (Bio-Oss) and implant dental implant system. Part II. Evaluation of deproteinized bovine bone (Bio-Oss) and implant surface. Acta Medica (Hradec Kralove) 2002; 45(4):167–71.

[51] Majorana C, Redemagni M, Rabagliati M, et al. Treatment of maxillary ridge resorption by sinus augmentation with iliac cancellous bone, anorganic bovine bone, and endosseous implants: a clinical and histologic report. Int J Oral Maxillofac Implants 2000; 15(6):873–8.

[52] Artzi Z, Nemcovsky CE, Dayan D. Bovine-HA spongiosa blocks and immediate implant placement in sinus augmentation procedures: histopathological and histomorphometric

observations on different histological stainings in 10 consecutive patients. Clin Oral Implants Res 2002;13(4):420–7.

[53] Hallman M, Lundgren S, Sennerby L. Histologic analysis of clinical biopsies taken 6 months and 3 years after maxillary sinus floor augmentation with 80% bovine hydroxyapatite and 20% autogenous bone mixed with fibrin glue. Clin Implant Dent Relat Res 2001; 3(2):87–96.

[54] Froum SJ, Tarnow DP, Wallace SS, et al. Sinus floor elevation using anorganic bovine bone matrix (OsteoGraf/N) with and without autogenous bone: a clinical, histologic, radiographic, and histomorphometric analysis. Part 2 of an ongoing prospective study. Int J Periodontics Restorative Dent 1998;18(6):528–43.

[55] Krauser JT, Rohrer MD, Wallace SS. Human histologic and histomorphometric analysis comparing OsteoGraf/N with PepGen P15 in the maxillary sinus elevation procedures: a case report. Implant Dent 2000;9(4):298–302.

[56] Bhatnagar RS, Qian JJ, Gough CA. The role in cell binding of a beta-0bend within the triple helical region in collagen alpha 1(I) chain: structural and biological evidence for conformational tautomerism on fiber surface. J Biomol Struct Dyn 1997;14(5):547–60.

[57] Bhatnagar RS, Qian JJ, Wedrchowska A, et al. Design of biomimetic habitats for tissue engineering with P-15, a synthetic peptide analogue of collagen. Tissue Eng 1999;5(1): 53–65.

[58] Thompson DM, Rohrer MD, Prasad HS. Comparison of bone grafting materials in human extraction sockets: clinical, histologic, and histomorphometric evaluations. Implant Dent 2006;15(1):89–96.

[59] Kubler A, Neugebauer J, Oh JH, et al. Growth and proliferation of human osteoblasts on different bone graft substitutes: an in vitro study. Implant Dent 2004;13(2):171–9.

[60] Turhani D, Item C, Thurner D, et al. Evidence of osteocalcin expression in osteoblast cells of mandibular origin growing on biomaterials with RT-PCR and SDS-PAGE/Western blotting [in German]. Mund Kiefer Gesichtschir 2003;7(5):294–300.

[61] Turhani D, Weissenbock M, Watzinger E, et al. In vitro study of adherent mandibular osteoblast-like cells on carrier materials. Int J Oral Maxillofac Surg 2005;34(5):543–50.

[62] Tabata M, Shimoda T, Sugihara K, et al. Osteoconductive and hemostatic properties of apatite formed on/in agarose gel as a bone-grafting material. J Boimed Mater Res B Appl Biomater 2003;67(2):680–8.

[63] Tabata M, Shimoda T, Sugihara K, et al. Apatite formed on/in agarose gel as a bone-grafting material in the treatment of periodontal infrabony defect. J Biomed Mater Res B Appl Biomater 2005;75(2):378–86.

[64] Mukherjee DP, Tunkle AS, Roberts RA, et al. An animal evaluation of a paste of chitosan glutamate and hydroxyapatite as a synthetic bone graft material. J Biomed Mater Res B Appl Biomater 2003;67(1):603–9.

[65] Silva RV, Camilli JA, Bertran CA, et al. The use of hydroxyapatite and autogenous cancellous bone grafts to repair bone defects in rats. Int J Oral Maxillofac Surg 2005;34(2): 178–84.

[66] Hsu FY, Tsai SW, Lan CW, et al. An in vivo study of a bone grafting material consisting of hydroxyapatite and reconstituted collagen. J Mater Sci Mater Med 2005;16(4):341–5.

[67] Thorwarth M, Schultze-Mosgau S, Kessler P, et al. Bone regeneration in osseous defects using a resorbable nanoparticular hydroxyapatite. J Oral Maxillofac Surg 2005;63(11): 1626–33.

[68] Baramki HG, Steffen T, Lander P, et al. The efficacy of interconnected porous hydroxyapatite in achieving posterolateral lumbar fusion in sheep. Spine 2000;25(9):1053–60.

[69] Mazor Z, Peleg M, Garg AK, et al. The use of hydroxyapatite bone cement for sinus floor augmentation with simultaneous implant placement in the atrophic maxilla: a report of 10 cases. J Periodontol 2000;71(7):1187–94.

[70] Goto T, Kojima T, Iijima T, et al. Resorption of synthetic porous hydroxyapatite and replacement by newly formed bone. J Orthop Sci 2001;6(5):444–7.

[71] Joosten U, Joist A, Frebel T, et al. The use of an in situ curing hydroxyapatite cement as an alternative to bone graft following removal of enchondroma of the hand. J Hand Surg [Br] 2000;25(3):288–91.

[72] Tuncer S, Yavuzer R, Isik I, et al. The fate of hydroxyapatite cement used for cranial contouring: histological evaluation of a case. J Craniofac Surg 2004;15(2):243–6.

[73] Briem D, Linhart W, Lehmann W, et al. Long-term outcomes after using porous hydroxyapatite ceramics (Endobon) for surgical management of fractures of the head of the tibia. Unfallchirurg 2002;105(2):128–33.

[74] Chiroff RT, White EW, Weber JN, et al. Tissue growth of replantiform implants. J Biomed Mater Res 1975;6:29–45.

[75] Roy DM, Linneham SK. Hydroxyapatite formed from coral skeletal carbonate by hydrothermal exchange. Nature 1974;247:220–32.

[76] Ewers R, Kasperk C, Simons B. A comparison of algae derived, coral derived and sintered hydroxyapatites with regard to physical properties and osteointegration [abstract]. Presented at the Materials Research Society Fall Meeting. Boston, September 17–21, 1987.

[77] Spassova-Tzekova E, Dimitriev Y, Evers R, et al. Properties and porosity of a physogenic apatite material produced by a biomimetic synthesis material. Biomaterials 2006, in press.

[78] Weissenboeck M, Stein E, Undt G, et al. Particle size of hydroxyapatite granules calcified from red algae affects the osteogenic potential of human mesenchymal stem cells in vitro. Cells Tissues Organs 2006;182(2):79–88.

[79] Klawitter JJ, Bagwell JG, Weinstein AM, et al. An evaluation of bone growth into porous high density polyethylene. J Biomed Mater Res 1976;10(2):311–23.

[80] Guillemin G, Meunier A, Dallant P, et al. Comparison of coral resorption and bone apposition with two natural corals of different porosities. J Biomed Mater Res 1989; 23:765–79.

[81] Wanschitz F, Gigl M, Wagner A, et al. Measurement of volume changes after sinus floor augmentation with a phycogenic hydroxyapatite. Int J Oral Maxillofac Implants 2004; 19:357–68.

[82] Leewenburgh S, Layrolle P, Barrere F, et al. Osteoclastic resorption of biomimetic calcium phosphate coatings in vitro. J Biomed Mater Res 2001;56:208–15.

[83] Demers C, Hamdy CR, Karin C, et al. Natural coral exoskeleton as a bone graft substitute: a review. Biomed Mater Eng 2002;12:15–35.

[84] Jammet P, Souyris F, Baldet P, et al. The effects of different porosities in coral implants: an experimental study. J Craniomaxillofac Surg 1994;22:103–8.

[85] Simunek A, Cierny M, Kopecka D, et al. The sinus lift with phycogenic bone substitute: a histomorphometric study. Clin Oral Implants Res 2005;16(3):342–8.

[86] Coughlin MJ, Grimes JS, Kennedy MP. Coralline hydroxyapatite bone graft substitute in hindfoot surgery. Foot Ankle Int 2006;27(1):19–22.

[87] Bojescul JA, Polly DW Jr, Kuklo TR, et al. Backfill for iliac-crest donor sites: a prospective, randomized study of coralline hydroxyapatite. Am J Orthop 2005;34(8):377–82.

[88] Tho KS, Krishnamoorthy S. Use of coral grafts in anterior interbony fusion of the rabbit spine. Ann Acad Med Singapore 1996;25(6):824–7.

[89] Hsu CJ, Chou WY, Teng HP, et al. Coralline hydroxyapatite and laminectomy-derived bone as adjuvant graft material for lumbar posterolateral fusions. J Neurosurg Spine 2005;3(4):271–5.

[90] El-Ghannam A. Bone reconstruction: from bioceramics to tissue engineering [review]. Expert Rev Med Devices 2005;2(1):87–101.

[91] Moreira-Gonzalez A, Lobocki C, Barakat K, et al. Evaluation of 45S5 bioactive glass combined as a bone substitute in the reconstruction of critical size calvarial defects in rabbits. J Craniofac Surg 2005;16(1):63–70.

[92] Griffon DJ, Dunlop DG, Howie CR, et al. Early dissolution of a morsellised impacted silicate-free bioactive glass in metaphyseal defects. J Biomed Mater Res 2001;58(6):638–44.

[93] Hall EE, Meffert RM, Hermann JS, et al. Comparison of bioactive glass to demineralized freeze-dried bone allograft in the treatment of intrabony defects around implants in the canine mandible. J Periodontol 1999;70(5):526–35.

[94] Wheeler DL, Eschbach EJ, Hoellrich RG, et al. Assessment of resorbable bioactive material for grafting of critical-size cancellous defects. J Orthop Res 2000;18(1):140–8.

[95] Cancian DC, Hochuli-Vieira E, Marcantonio RA, et al. Utilization of autogenous bone, bioactive glasses, and calcium phosphate cement in surgical mandibular bone defects in Cebus apella monkeys. Int J Oral Maxillofac Implants 2004;19(1):73–9.

[96] Lindfors NC, Tallroth K, Aho AJ. Bioactive glass as bone-graft substitute for posterior spinal fusion in rabbit. J Biomed Mater Res 2002;63(2):237–44.

[97] Lindfors NC, Aho AJ. Tissue response to bioactive glass and autogenous bone in the rabbit spine. Eur Spine J 2000;9(1):30–5.

[98] Froum S, Cho SC, Rosenberg E, et al. Histological comparison of healing extraction sockets implanted with bioactive glass or demineralized freeze-dried bone allograft: a pilot study. J Periodontol 2002;73(1):94–102.

[99] Furusawa T, Mizunuma K. Osteoconductive properties and efficacy of resorbable bioactive glass as a bone-grafting material. Implant Dent 1997;6(2):93–101.

[100] Turunen T, Peltola J, Yli-Urpo A, et al. Bioactive glass granules as a bone adjunctive material in maxillary sinus floor augmentation. Clin Oral Implants Res 2004;15(2):135–41.

[101] Tadjoedin ES, de Lange GL, Lyaruu DM, et al. High concentrations of bioactive glass material (BioGran) vs. autogenous bone for sinus floor elevation. Clin Oral Implants Res 2002; 13(4):428–36.

[102] Cordioli G, Mazzocco C, Schepers E, et al. Maxillary sinus floor augmentation using bioactive glass granules and autogenous bone with simultaneous implant placement: clinical and histological findings. Clin Oral Implants Res 2001;12(3):270–8.

[103] Tadjoedin ES, de Lange GL, Holzmann PJ, et al. Histological observations on biopsies harvested following sinus floor elevation using a bioactive glass material of narrow size range. Clin Oral Implants Res 2000;11(4):334–44.

[104] Butz SJ, Huys LW. Long-term success of sinus augmentation using a synthetic alloplast: a 20 patients, 7 years clinical report. Implant Dent 2005;14(1):36–42.

[105] Wikipedia. Available at: http://en.wikipedia.org/wiki/tricalcium-phosphate. Accessed 2006.

[106] Pietrzak WS, Ronk R. Calcium sulfate bone void filler: a review and a look ahead. J Craniofac Surg 2000;11(4):327–33.

[107] Maragos P, Bissada NF, Wang R, et al. Comparison of three methods using calcium sulfate as a graft/barrier material for the treatment of Class II mandibular molar furcation defects. Int J Periodontics Restorative Dent 2002;22(5):493–501.

[108] Borrelli J Jr, Prickett WD, Ricci WM. Treatment of nonunions and osseous defects with bone graft and calcium sulfate. Clin Orthop Relat Res 2003;(411):245–54.

[109] Moore RM, Graves SE, Gain GI. Synthetic bone graft substitute. ANZ J Surg 2001;71: 354–61.

[110] Coetzee AS. Regeneration of bone in the presence of calcium sulphate. Arch Orolaryngol 1980;106:405–9.

[111] Herron S, Thordarson DB, Winet H, et al. Ingrowth of bone into absorbable bone cement: an in vivo microscopic evaluation. Am J Orthop 2003;32(12):581–4.

[112] Blokhuis TJ, Wippermann BW, den Boer FC, et al. Resorbable calcium phosphate particles as a carrier material for bone marrow in an ovine segmental defect. J Biomed Mater Res 2000;51(3):369–75.

[113] Linhart W, Briem D, Schmitz ND, et al. Treatment of metaphyseal bone defects after fractures of the distal radius: medium-term results using a calcium-phosphate cement (BIOBON). Unfallchirurg 2003;106(8):618–24.

[114] Aybar B, Bilir A, Akcakaya H, et al. Effects of tricalcium phosphate bone graft materials on primary cultures of osteoblast cells in vitro. Clin Oral Implants Res 2004;15(1):119–25.

[115] Fredericks DC, Bobst JA, Petersen EB, et al. Cellular interactions and bone healing responses to a novel porous tricalcium phosphate bone graft material. Orthopedics 2004; 27(1 Suppl):s167–73.

[116] Artzi Z, Weinreb M, Givol N, et al. Biomaterial resorption rate and healing site morphology of inorganic bovine bone and beta-tricalcium phosphate in the canine: a 24-month longitudinal histologic study and morphometric analysis. Int J Oral Maxillofac Implants 2004; 19(3):357–68.

[117] Szabo G, Suba Z, Hrabak K, et al. Autogenous bone versus beta-tricalcium phosphate graft alone for bilateral sinus elevations (2- and 3-dimensional computed tomographic, histologic, and histomorphometric evaluations): preliminary results. Int J Oral Maxillofac Implants 2001;16(5):681–92.

[118] Suba Z, Hrabak K, Huys L, et al. Histologic and histomorphometric study of bone regeneration induced by beta-tricalcium phosphate (multicenter study). Orv Hetil 2004;145(27): 1431–7.

[119] Szabo G, Huy L, Coulthard P, et al. A prospective multicenter randomized clinical trial of autogenous bone versus beta-tricalcium phosphate graft along for bilateral sinus elevation: histologic and histomorphometric evaluation. Int J Oral Maxillofac Implants 2005;20(3): 371–81.

[120] Nemeth Z, Suba Z, Hrabak K, et al. Autogenous bone versus beta-tricalcium phosphate graft alone for bilateral sinus evaluations (2-3D CT, histologic and histomorphometric evaluations). Orv Hetil 2002;143(25):1533–8.

[121] Velich N, Nemeth Z, Toth C, et al. Long-term results with different bone substitutes used for sinus floor elevation. J Craniofac Surg 2004;14(1):38–41.

[122] Scher EL, Day RB, Speight PM. New bone formation after a sinus lift procedure using demineralized freeze-dried bone and tricalcium phosphate. Implant Dent 1999;8(1): 49–53.

[123] Anker CJ, Holdridge SP, Baird B, et al. Ultraporous beta-tricalcium phosphate is well incorporated in small cavitary defects. Clin Orthop Relat Res 2005;(434):251–7.

[124] Pittner MF, Alaster MM, Beck SC, et al. Multilineage potential of adult human mesenchymal stem cells. Science 1999;284(5411):143–7.

[125] Forbes SJ, Poulsom R, Wright NA. Hepatic and renal differentiation from blood-borne stem cells. Gene Ther 2002;9(10):625–30.

[126] Pittenger MF, Mosca JD, McIntosh KR. Human mesenchymal stem cells: progenitor cell for cartilage, bone, fat and stroma. Curr Top Microbiol Immunol 2000;251:3–11.

[127] De Ugarte DA, Kouki M, Elbarbari A, et al. Comparison of multi-lineage cells from human adipose tissue and bone marrow. Cells Tissues Organs 2003;174(3):101–9.

[128] Banfi A, et al. Proliferation kinetics and differentiation potential of ex vivo expanded human bone marrow stromal cells: implications for their use in cell therapy. Exp Hematol 2000;28(2):707–15.

[129] Wagers AJ, Weissman IL. Plasticity of adult stem cells. Cell 2004;116(5):639–48.

[130] Zuk PA, Zhu M, Mizuno H, et al. Multilineage cells from human adipose tissue: implications for cell-based therapies. Tissue Eng 2001;7(2):211–28.

[131] Hidemi H, Masato S, Kazunori M, et al. Osteogenic potential of human adipose tissue derived stromal cells as an alternative stem cell source. Cells, Tissues, Organs 2004;178(1): 2–12.

[132] Hicok KC, du Laney TV, Zhou YS, et al. Human adipose-derived adult stem cells produce osteoid in vivo. Tissue Eng 2004;10(3–4):371–80.

[133] Sato M, Ochi T, Nakase T, et al. Mechanical tension-stress induces expression of bone morphogenetic protein (BMP)-2 and BMP-4, but not BMP-6, BMP-7, and GDF-5 mRNA, during distraction osteogenesis. J Bone Miner Res 1999;14(7):1084–95.

[134] Campisi P, Hamdy RC, Lauzier D, et al. Expression of bone morphogenetic proteins during mandibular distraction osteogenesis. Plst Reconstr Surg 2003;111(1):201–8 [discussion: 209–10].

[135] Saadeh PB, Khosia RK, Mehrara BJ, et al. Repair of a critical size defect in the rat mandible using allogenic type I collagen. J Craniofac Surg 2001;12(6):573–9.

[136] Seol YJ, Lee JY, Park YJ, et al. Chitosan sponges as tissue engineering scaffolds for bone formation. Biotechnol Lett 2004;26(13):1037–41.

[137] Bumgardner JD, Wiser R, Gerard PD, et al. Chitosan: potential use as a bioactive coating for orthopaedic and craniofacial/dental implant. J Biomater Sci Polym Ed 2003;14(15): 423–38.

[138] Solchaga LA, Dennis JE, Goldberg VM, et al. Treatment of osteochondral defects with autologous bone marrow in a hyaluronan-based delivery vehicle. Tissue Eng 2002;8(2): 333–47.

[139] Cao Y, Vacanti JP, Paige KT, et al. Transplantation of chondrocytes utilizing a polymer-cell construct to produce tissue-engineered cartilage in the shape of a human ear. Plast Reconstr Surg 1997;100:297–302 [discussion: 3–4].

[140] Behravesh E, Yasko AW, Engel PS, et al. Synthetic biodegradable polymers for orthopaedic applications. Clin Orthop Relat Res 1999;367(Suppl):S118–29.

[141] Lendlein A, Langer R. Biodegradable, elastic shape-memory polyers for potential biomedical applications. Science 2002;296:2673–6.

[142] Gunatillake PA, Adhikari R. Biodegradable synthetic polymers for tissue engineering. Eur Cell Mater 2003;5:1–16.

ELSEVIER
SAUNDERS

Dent Clin N Am 51 (2007) 747–760

THE DENTAL
CLINICS
OF NORTH AMERICA

Biocompatibility of Dental Materials

Kenneth R. St. John, PhD

Department of Biomedical Materials Science, University of Mississippi Medical Center School of Dentistry, 2500 North State Street, Jackson 39216, USA

For more than 2000 years, humans have attempted to improve life through the use of materials and devices of nonhuman origin as prosthetic devices and restorative materials in contact with tissues in the oral and maxillofacial environments [1]. Initially, the patient or someone providing care might use whatever materials were close at hand to make repairs and prosthetics. Before 400BC, the Etruscans were fabricating bridges and partial dentures using gold combined with animal or extracted human teeth. As communications improved and humans became more mobile and more urbanized, dentists and health care providers realized that some materials were more successful than others when used in contact with oral and maxillofacial tissues. At about the same time, researchers in other fields of medicine were also realizing that the tissue response to some materials was more favorable than the response to other materials. Some of the first publications to look at the evaluation of the tissue response to dental materials were those of Autian and his colleagues [2–6] in the early 1970s, and an early review article was published in 1971 [7].

Depending on how biocompatibility is defined, the term may include adverse effects of a material on tissues and physiologic systems, adverse effects of the physiologic environment on the material, or a combination of the two, such as an adverse tissue response to the products of material degradation caused by physiologic exposure. The biocompatibility of a material depends upon the type of material, where it is placed, and the function it is expected to perform. Therefore, a material cannot be biocompatible but it does elicit an acceptable tissue response when tested or used in a specific tissue or category of tissue under certain conditions, including the health status of the patient [8].

Areas of biocompatibility concern

The oral and maxillofacial environment is complex and varied, with different requirements and different biocompatibility issues depending on the

E-mail address: kstjohn@sod.umsmed.edu

specific use. Other than fully implanted materials, exposure includes exposure to saliva, foodstuffs, bacteria, and the products of interactions between components of the environment. These exposures place severe requirements on the performance of the device components and may have requirements unique to this environment. Although most sites in the body in which biomedical materials may be placed have a relatively constant temperature and chemical composition (in the absence of infection or inflammation), the oral environment exhibits extremes of temperature, pH, and chemical composition of food. The extremes of temperature from that of ice cream ($0°C$) to hot coffee ($90°C$) may lead to compatibility problems, such as thermal expansion, changes in mechanical properties, or failure of bonding. The pH in the microenvironment around dental caries–causing bacteria may be as low as 2.2 [9]. The pH of gastric secretions is 1.0 to 3.5 [10], and the pH of the acid produced in the stomach is 0.8. [10]. The exposure of intraoral materials to gastric contents because of reflux or regurgitation as a result of medical conditions or bulimia presents a special biocompatibility challenge that, although not the normal physiologic condition, may require consideration under some circumstances.

When caries are removed from a tooth, the cavity created may provide the opportunity for chemical components or degradation products of dental materials to migrate to the pulp chamber of the tooth, meaning that it is necessary to be concerned about the possible toxic effects on blood, capillary tissues, and neurons and potential problems with the tissues in the mouth. If there is a possible problem with the contact of certain materials with the contacts of the pulp chamber, then appropriate precautions must be taken to isolate the restorative material, such as the use of cavity liners.

In general, the most benign tissue response seen to materials placed within living tissues is the formation of a fibrous tissue capsule around the material, walling it off from the physiologic environment. The thickness of this capsule is sometimes used as one indicator of the acceptability of the material, because a thicker capsule suggests that the body is continuing to produce additional fibrous tissue in response to a continuing irritant that has not yet been minimized by the capsule that has formed. There are exceptions to the formation of a fibrous tissue capsule, in which bone may be formed directly on the surface of a material without any capsule. Certain metals and ceramics exhibit this characteristic.

Restorative materials

Restorative materials include those used for replacing carious tissue within the tooth structure, such as inlays and onlays, crowns, bridges, partial dentures, and full dentures. Many of the materials used to fill cavities are normally not placed into direct contact with tissues other than dentin and enamel. They are subject to corrosion, wear, and leaching of constituent chemicals [11]. If a curing reaction is involved in placement, an exotherm may occur, monomers or other chemicals may be released, or the raw materials may leach through the dentin tubules and into the pulp chamber and come into contact with blood and nerve tissue. Additionally, materials used in endodontic therapy must come into contact with the pulp space and its contents, and it may leak into periapical tissues, creating additional concerns beyond those for materials intended to restore the crown morphology [12,13]. When used in contact with gingiva or the tissue lining the mouth, additional testing for tissue response may be necessary, and the possibilities for problems caused by direct contact increase.

Amalgam

The biocompatibility of amalgam, a product of the reaction of liquid mercury with silver and other metals, has been the subject of controversy for many years. There has been a concern that the mercury used in the reaction may leach out of the restoration as a result of unreacted material, dissolution in saliva, or corrosion reactions. It is known that mercury exists inorganically as the metal or in one of two charge states and in an organic form (methyl mercury). When present as methyl mercury, it is known to be highly toxic. Methyl mercury has been responsible for toxic reactions in the hat industry, in environmental disasters, and through consumption of seafood. Mercury in vapor form is easily taken up by the body. The mercury present in an amalgam reaction exists in the metallic form and is not easily absorbed from the digestive system if swallowed. It is completely bound up with the other metals present in the amalgam because the reaction is a chemical one that combines it with the metals to form an alloy.

Studies reviewed by the US Public Health Service and the Food and Drug Administration suggest that based on available evidence, there is no proof of any mercury toxicity from dental amalgam to the patient, other than in cases of allergy [14–17]. A study published in the *New England Journal of Medicine* [18] concluded that there is no clear evidence for the removal of amalgams and that the evidence is open to wide interpretation. The authors of two reviews published in Europe concluded, "According to the conclusions of independent evaluations from different state health agencies, the release of mercury from dental amalgam does not present any nonacceptable risk to the general population" [19] and "...there is little evidence of a correlation between amalgam restorations and adverse neurological or neuropsychological effects...That said, additional studies are needed to strengthen the case" [20]. Two studies reported on amalgam use in children and examined a total of 520 children who received amalgam randomly matched against 521 who received composite restorations. One study concluded that "...there is no reason to discontinue the use of mercury amalgam as the standard of care for caries in posterior teeth" [21]. The other concluded that "...amalgam should remain a viable clinical option in dental restorative treatment" [22].

Polymeric materials and composites

Many restorative materials other than amalgam are compounds that are polymerized or otherwise reacted in the prepared tooth cavity at the time of placement [23–25]. These materials consist of monomers, fillers, initiators, accelerators, and additives that are combined through some type of a curing reaction [11,26–29]. If the proportions of the different components are not correct or if the curing reactions are not carried to completion, some or all of the components may be available to become dissolved in saliva, pass through tubules into the pulp chamber, or otherwise be released. Some monomer also may be released before curing occurs or during curing. Initiators and accelerators, depending on the type of curing reaction, may cause polymerization to occur or be accelerated without actually becoming a part of the polymer chain, which leads to the possibility that they may be free to diffuse out of the material and come into contact with tissues. In the same way, additives such as plasticizers act to change the mechanical properties of the final product but are not necessarily bound up in the constituent polymers.

Metallic materials

When metals and alloys are used in dentistry, there is the opportunity for adverse reactions caused by the release of metal ions or other products of the interaction between the physiologic environment and the metals [30]. Except for certain noble metals, pure metals and alloys used in dentistry derive biocompatibility from the formation of a protective layer on the surface called a passive film, which is an oxide of one or more of the components of the alloy [11,31,32]. These films are products of an oxidative (corrosive) reaction that reduces the corrosion rate by several orders of magnitude and essentially prevents further corrosion once the passive layer is formed. Because this layer is protective, anything that disturbs the layer can lead to either a brief period of repassivation or, under the wrong conditions, failure to protect the underlying metal from corrosion. Contact between two different metals in the mouth or changes in the temperature or pH in the mouth can cause breakdown in protection and can, in the case of dissimilar metals, lead to galvanic corrosion. Even when the passive film is intact, the corrosion rate is not zero—just very small. Metal ions are being released at slow rates, but the body can have adverse reactions to those ions. There may be local toxic responses, systemic changes in metabolic processes, or an allergic response to certain metal ions [11,33–36]. Although uncommon, the metal most frequently responsible for an allergic response is nickel, which is present in most stainless steels, most cobalt/chromium alloys, nickel-titanium alloys, and nickel-chromium alloys. If an adverse allergic response occurs, little can be done other than to exchange the metal component for one that does not contain nickel.

Another way that an adverse response can occur is if corrosion produces particles of corrosive product, which can induce the same type of tissue response that may result from the formation of wear particles (see later discussion).

One positive aspect of the use of metals in implant surgery is that titanium and its alloys (and potentially other metals) have caused bone to attach directly to the metal without any intervening soft tissue capsule [31,32,37]. This occurrence is considered to be evidence of superior biocompatibility of titanium and is the basis for many of the applications of titanium in dentistry. It is likely that the favorable response may be to the TiO$_2$ passive film that is present on the surface and not to the titanium itself. Recently, there has been some caution expressed that, under certain conditions of chemical exposure and pH in the oral environment, titanium and its alloys may not exhibit the high corrosion resistance and stable passive film that has been reported previously [38].

Ceramic materials

The tissue response to ceramic materials used in surgery falls into two basic categories: (1) porcelains and other hard ceramics used in crowns, inlays, and onlays and (2) ceramics that are intended to react with surrounding tissues. It is also important to note that the passive films that form on metals to protect them from corrosion are ceramic in nature and are the actual interface being presented to tissue on metals. Ceramics of the first type would seem to be insoluble and, with (theoretically) little or no chemical being released from them and little opportunity for tissue to respond, there should be little concern with their biocompatibility. Not as much attention has been applied to their testing [11,39]. Some researchers have found that this assumption may not be true [40]. In cell culture experiments, some ceramics were found to cause little suppression of mitochondria activity, some were found to be initially toxic, but that toxicity declined after an artificial aging process, one was extremely cytotoxic and became toxic again after repolishing, and one did not regain its toxicity with repolishing. The conclusion was that the aging process was removing cytotoxic chemicals from the ceramics but that the leaching was only from the surface in some cases while being from the bulk of the material in others. In reviewing reports of biocompatibility testing, it is important to review the condition of the materials being tested. In the referenced study, the ceramics that were not cytotoxic (feldspathic veneer porcelains) were fired before testing, but the other three materials tested were processed by pressing into molds according to manufacturer's instructions but had not been subjected to the final sintering treatment. It is possible that the sintering process would have bound up the toxic species into the bulk and prevented a tissue response.

The other class of tissue responses to ceramics concerns ceramics that are intended to interact with the surrounding tissues. In general, these materials do not have the necessary mechanical properties for use in crowns and other restorations but undergo at least a small amount of dissolution at the surface and are composed of compounds that contain calcium and phosphorus, two of the elements that comprise the mineral content of bone. Bioglass and calcium phosphate ceramics, such as hydroxyapatite and tricalcium phosphate, interact with surrounding bone to form a bond between the material and the tissue that can be stronger than either the bone or the material itself [41–44]. In a process called osteointegration, the materials become integrated into the bone as it repairs itself and may reside permanently within the healed bone, although some are dissolved or resorbed and replaced by new bone [45]. These materials are intentionally reactive with bone but are recognized and incorporated as if they were bone.

Wear

Whenever two surfaces experience relative movement, there is the opportunity for wear and the formation of wear particles surrounding the site where wear is occurring. The tissue response to small particles of a material can be different to that for the bulk material. Particles small enough to be phagocytized by cells can induce a cascade of tissue responses and the release of cellular mediators, which may then act as positive reinforcers to the process and result in significant tissue responses [46,47]. Although not exactly the result of wear, particles of material may be released into tissues because of corrosion, polishing and finishing operations, or inadvertent loss of a small piece of the material during other dental procedures, such as placement or removal of a dental dam or removal of impression material from the mouth. As a particle is phagocytized, it enters the same defensive process that the body would use to defend itself from a cellular attacker, such as a bacterium. Although the engulfment of a bacterium can result in the death of the attacker and the defender cell, in the case of biomaterials the defender cell may die and release the offending particle back into the surrounding tissue intact. These cells may release chemical signaling compounds to cause recruiting of additional defender cells. If the particles are not dissolved in the process or otherwise removed from the tissues, the same particles can be repeatedly phagocytized and released, increasing the levels of chemical mediators in the tissues. These chemicals themselves can have an adverse effect on the tissues by activating or deactivating cells, such as fibroblasts, osteoblasts, and osteoclasts [48,49].

Most of the research that examines the physiologic consequences of wear has centered on orthopedic devices because the wear occurs within an enclosed space and clinical failures have been seen in that environment. In dental and maxillofacial applications, the wear of restorative materials has less potential for the particles to enter the tissues, because wear particles and particles produced during placement and finishing are more likely to be ingested or removed by rinsing and suction. The potential exists for particles to enter periodontal pockets, and the wear of temporomandibular joint prostheses has been shown to produce problems similar to those from the wear of total joint prostheses in orthopedic surgery [50].

The amount of wear that may occur between two surfaces subjected to loads while undergoing relative motion can be related to several different factors, but the amount of frictional forces applied at the interface is directly proportional to the load being applied perpendicular to the wearing surfaces. The forces present at occlusal surfaces during chewing and the forces present at the temporomandibular joint can be high. The force on molars can be as high as 800 to 900 N [51,52], so wear forces being generated can be significant. Because of the lever action of the temporomandibular joint, the forces dissipated through the joint can be different than forces experienced at the occlusal surfaces.

Test methods

Testing for biocompatibility depends on the actual site of use and the duration of exposure. Materials that are used for manufacturing dental instruments and other associated products do not have to exhibit the same compatibility as materials that are placed permanently into the tooth structure or the pulp chamber, used as implants into bone or soft tissues, or used in dentures and dental and orthodontic appliances. Testing is usually conducted sequentially, with shorter term, in vitro, or less expensive screening testing being performed before more extensive and time-consuming testing that involves the use of animals. If a material is shown to have a biocompatibility problem based on initial studies, it may be possible to eliminate it from consideration for further testing for certain applications. Review of published biocompatibility studies can give clues about which materials may be most suitable or show that testing is not necessary if a particular material already has been tested thoroughly and shown to be acceptable for the intended application. In 1985, a textbook of testing methods and their applicability and conduct was published, and a more recent publication provides additional guidance and discussion of testing methods [8,53]. These protocols and methods of interpretation may be used to augment the information given in the national and international standards.

Although most of the biocompatibility concerns and testing methods discussed in this article have been in use for more than 40 years, new issues and new testing possibilities must be considered as dental materials continue to develop. Attempts have been made to evaluate the response of cells to medical materials at the cellular and subcellular levels. Currently, investigators look at what happens adjacent to materials rather than determine why a particular response is seen. Instead of looking at the tissue reaction by observation of cell proliferation or death in contact with materials, new efforts focus on trying to determine why the observed response occurs. If researchers can determine how cellular membrane properties change or what chemical mediators may be released or taken up at the material interface, it may be possible to determine which material properties are responsible for the reactions and allow the design of materials that have surface properties or chemical contents to take advantage of these cellular and subcellular responses [54]. The advent of tissue-engineered materials may allow the creation of tissue-based solutions to some dental problems, giving rise to new concerns for biocompatibility testing.

Cell culture testing

A common first step in the evaluation of a new material is placing the material or an extract of the material into a suitable laboratory cell culture and observing any changes in the cells over a period of hours to a few days [55]. These tests are not normally performed on cultures of cells actually taken from the oral environment but, more commonly, are conducted using established cell lines that are commercially available, which allows comparison of testing performed for different materials using nearly identical cloned cells. These cells may be fibroblasts, macrophages, or other types of cells. The cells are placed into a culture dish or multi-well culture array and allowed to grow and reproduce under controlled conditions until the bottom of the container is covered with a uniform single layer of cells. The material sample or a fluid extract of the material is added to the culture, and the containers are returned to the incubator for up to 3 days. The cultures are then examined under the microscope, and changes in the cells or regions of cell death are recorded and scored to produce a final biocompatibility score. These test results are evaluated and combined with knowledge of the intended application, and the suitability of the material is determined. These tests typically do not have a specific passing score but are interpreted in comparison with positive and negative controls whose tissue responses in vivo are known. The negative control is generally accepted as a suitable material for the intended application, and the positive control is known to elicit a strong toxic response.

Mutagenicity testing

The possibility that long-term exposure to a material may lead to neoplastic changes in adjacent cells is a concern for any material used in medicine. Most materials are known to be acceptable based on a history of use, but changes in formulations and the development of new materials occasionally necessitate testing. As described later, conducting carcinogenicity studies is expensive and time consuming. In vitro and small animal in vivo mutagenicity studies allow screening of materials early in development and reduce the use of research animals. Mutagenicity studies (also called genotoxicity studies) involve looking for changes in cells and cellular DNA in the forward or reverse directions. In forward mutation studies, normal cells are exposed to the test material and the resultant cells or animal tissues are evaluated for signs of mutation. Detecting changes in small numbers of cells can be problematic, and reverse mutation studies are frequently chosen. In reverse mutation studies, studies are performed on cells that are abnormal and have a characteristic not present in normal cells, such as the requirement for a particular chemical entity for growth that normal cells do not require. Studies are performed in the presence and absence of the vital chemical, and if growth occurs without the presence of the chemical, then repair of the DNA has occurred as a result of exposure to the material. Changes in cellular DNA in either direction indicate mutagenic potential for the material.

Short-term injection or implantation studies

Several different tests may be conducted to provide information on effects of relatively short-term exposure to materials or their extracts. These tests include systemic injection of an extract for toxicity, intracutaneous injection for irritation, and short-term implant studies. These studies allow screening of materials for periods as short as 24 hours and as long as 90 days to ascertain the systemic and local tissue response to the materials. The end results of these tests are primarily pathologic interpretations of tissue samples or observations of the overall health of the animals. Injection studies are concluded after 72 hours, whereas implantation studies assess tissue response for up to 90 days. These studies allow screening out of candidate materials that may not be suitable for further testing.

Irritation, sensitization, and immunotoxicity studies

Certain materials have the potential to cause local inflammation of tissues—even those not penetrated by the material—or the development of a systemic immune response. Tests determine whether a test animal will develop tissue response to contact with the material with repeated exposures. Much more severe would be the development of an immune response not confined to the contact area. One frequently encountered response is the inflammation of tissues in contact with stainless steel caused by sensitization to nickel, a component of the alloy. Many applications in the oral cavity involve long-term contact with the gingiva or mucous membranes, and persons who have sensitivity to a particular material should receive a substitute material. These tests measure the potential for the development of a response in vitro or in animals but do not determine whether specific patients should avoid a specific material.

Long-term implantation studies

Long-term studies continue for several years or, in some cases, for the life of the experimental animals. Tests may be conducted using test coupons of a material implanted into an appropriate animal site with respect to the intended use or may involve performing the actual clinical procedures with the material in larger animals, such as dogs, sheep, goats, or primates. One concern that may be raised with some of the implantation studies is determining the proper interpretation of the results [56]. The materials are left in place for a period of 1 or 2 years with intermediate sampling times. Once the experiment is completed for a particular sampling interval, all organs of the experimental animal are analyzed to look for toxic effects or other problems and perform an analysis of the implant site or site of placement.

A special case of long-term implantation studies involves the lifetime bioassay performed for investigation of carcinogenicity. This study is usually performed in several hundred rats and mice to look for differences in tumor formation as a result of exposure to the test material. The animals are allowed to live out their total life span, and the number, location, and characteristics of any tumors are investigated and recorded. Because a positive control is normally not used, it is necessary to use animal strains that are known to produce a certain number and type of tumors during aging without any exposure to a test material. This development allows for a comparison between the normal processes and those after exposure to the test material to determine whether there are differences in incidence, type, or location of tumors.

Standardization

In an effort to make the testing of dental materials for biocompatibility more uniform within individual countries and around the world, standards development groups within several organizations have issued documents specifying or recommending the testing that should be performed to determine the suitability of new and existing materials in the oral and maxillofacial environment [57,58]. In addition to the standards documents specific to dental materials, an additional ISO standard [59] and its related standards are referenced in the standard for dental materials; another similar document that has applicability to all types of medical materials, including dental materials, is available [60]. Many issues are related to the selection of appropriate test methodology, among them the anticipated site of implantation or use, the types of tissues with which the material is in contact, and the duration of tissue exposure to the material or its associated byproducts. Each of the referenced testing standards categorizes materials according to type of tissue contact and site of contact. All standards but the American Dental Association document also separate testing requirements by duration of contact. In the case of the American Dental Association practice, the types of dental materials are specifically called out and the duration of exposure is inherent in the description.

Regulations

In the United States, new medical products and devices are subject to regulation and approval by the US Food and Drug Administration, and similar organizations and rules exist in many other countries around the world. The US Food and Drug Administration issues guidelines for the types of testing that may be required and reported as a part of the approval process before devices may be placed into use, some of which apply to dental materials. Eight guidance documents have been issued in final form [61–68], and the document for labeling of amalgam is still in draft form for public comment [69]. Documents that require the reporting of biocompatibility testing that was performed reference the ISO standards [58,59], and the newer ones (since 2002) suggest their use instead of the American Dental Association standard [57]. whereas older documents suggest reference to the American Dental Association document for test methodology. References to published test methods are also included in the two international test matrix documents [59,60].

Summary

Although materials used in dentistry and oral surgery may not be subject to some of the biocompatibility challenges faced by materials used in other medical specialties, some of the requirements are unique because of the nature and anatomy of the tissues and structures being supported or reconstructed and because of the high loads that may be placed on them. Many of the criteria for testing and validating the biocompatibility of new materials are similar to those for materials used in other sites in the body. The specialized requirements for some aspects of dental material use have resulted in specialized protocols being developed for testing.

With the long history of use of many materials in dental surgery, biocompatibility concerns are not as great a concern as other issues, such as long-term degradation, mechanical strength problems, and prevention of secondary caries. It is important, however, not to forget that the potential exists for adverse tissue responses to synthetic materials used in repair, augmentation, and repair of natural tissue structures.

As new materials and repair techniques become available and the sophistication of cell-level and subcellular response evaluations increases, the concerns to be addressed and the methods to be used may change. The advent of tissue-engineered medical products may mean that new questions must be addressed.

References

[1] Bremner MDK. The Greeks, Etruscan, and Romans. In: The story of dentistry from the dawn of civilization to the present: with special emphasis on the American scene. Brooklyn (NY): Dental Items of Interest Publishing Company; 1954. p. 45–57.

[2] Autian J. The use of rabbit implants and tissue culture tests for the evaluation of dental materials. Int Dent J 1970;20(3):481–90.

[3] Powell D, Lawrence WH, Turner J, et al. Development of a toxicity evaluation program for dental materials and products. I. Screening for irritant responses. J Biomed Mater Res 1970; 4(4):583–96.

[4] Lawrence WH, Malik M, Autian J. Development of a toxicity evaluation program for dental materials and products. II. Screening for systemic toxicity. J Biomed Mater Res 1974;8(1): 11–34.

[5] Autian J. General and screening tests for dental materials. Int Dent J 1974;24(2):235–50.

[6] Autian J. A need for a more comprehensive testing program for dental implants. Oral Implantol 1974;5(1):9–23.

[7] Zeines V. The effect of restorative materials on the periodontal tissue: a review of the literature. NY J Dent 1971;41(3):101–5.

[8] Wataha JC. Principles of biocompatibility for dental practitioners. J Prosthet Dent 2001; 86(2):203–9.

[9] Badet MC, Richard B, Dorignac G. An in vitro study of the pH-lowering potential of salivary lactobacilli associated with dental caries. J Appl Microbiol 2001;90(6): 1015–8.

[10] Guyton AC, Hall JE. Textbook of medical physiology. 9th edition. Philadelphia: W.B. Saunders; 1996. p. 386, 817.

[11] Lygre H. Prosthodontic biomaterials and adverse reactions: a critical review of the clinical and research literature. Acta Odontol Scand 2002;60(1):1–9.

[12] Haumann CHJ, Love RM. Biocompatibility of dental materials used in contemporary endodontic surgery: a review. Part 1. Intracanal Drugs and Substances. Int Endodont J 2003; 36(2):75–85.

[13] Haumann CHJ, Love RM. Biocompatibility of dental materials used in contemporary endodontic surgery: a review. Part 2. Root-canal-filling materials. Int Endodont J 2003;36(3): 147–60.

[14] Public Health Service. Dental amalgam: a scientific review and recommended public health service strategy for research, education and regulation. Available at: http://www.health.gov/environment/amalgam1/ct.htm. Accessed June 29, 2006.

[15] Public Health Service. Dental amalgam and alternative restorative materials. USPHS risk management strategy: a status update. Available at: http://www.health.gov/environment/amalgam2/contents.html. Accessed July 25, 2006.

[16] US Food and Drug Administration. Consumer update: dental amalgams. Available at: http://www.fda.gov/cdrh/consumer/amalgams.html. Accessed July 25, 2006.

[17] Centers for Disease Control and Prevention. Fact sheet: dental amalgam use and benefits. Available at: http://www.cdc.gov/OralHealth/factsheets/amalgam.htm. Accessed July 25, 2006.

[18] Clarkson TW, Magos L, Myers GJ. Current concepts: the toxicology of mercury: current exposures and clinical manifestations. N Engl J Med 2003;349(18):1731–7.

[19] Ekstrand J, Björkman L, Edlund C, et al. Toxicological aspects on the release and systemic update of mercury from dental amalgam. Eur J Oral Sci 1998;106(2 Pt 2):678–86.

[20] Mitchell RJ, Osborne PB, Haubenreich JE. Dental amalgam restorations: daily mercury dose and biocompatibility. J Long Term Eff Med Implants 2005;15(6):709–21.

[21] Bellinger DC, Trachtenberg F, Barregard L, et al. Neuropsychological and renal effects of dental amalgam in children: a randomized clinical trial. JAMA 2006;295(15):1775–83.

[22] DeRouen TA, Martin MD, Leroux BG, et al. Neurobehavioral effects of dental amalgam in children: a randomized clinical trial. JAMA 2006;295(15):1784–92.

[23] Frazer RQ, Byron RT, Osborne PB, et al. PMMA: an essential material in medicine and dentistry. J Long Term Eff Med Implants 2005;15(6):629–39.

[24] Stein PS, Sullivan J, Haubenreich JE, et al. Composite resin in medicine and dentistry. J Long Term Eff Med Implants 2005;15(6):641–54.

[25] Kavorick RE, Haubenreich JE, Gore D. Glass ionomer cements: a review of composition, chemistry, and biocompatibility as a dental and medical implant material. J Long Term Eff Med Implants 2005;15(6):655–71.

[26] Hume WR, Gerzina TM. Bioavailability of components of resin-based materials which are applied to teeth. Crit Rev Oral Biol Med 1996;7(2):172–9.

[27] Guertsen W. Substances released from dental resin composites and glass ionomer cements. Eur J Oral Sci 1998;106(2 Pt 2):687–95.

[28] Schmalz G. The biocompatibility of non-amalgam dental filling materials. Eur J Oral Sci 1998;106(2 Pt 2):696–706.

[29] Geurtsen W. Biocompatibility of resin-modified filling materials. Crit Rev Oral Biol Med 2000;11(3):333–55.

[30] Gore DR, Frazer RQ, Kovarik RE, et al. Vitallium. J Long Term Eff Med Implants 2005; 15(6):673–86.

[31] Kasemo B, Lausmaa J. Metal selection and surface characteristics. In: Brånemark P-I, Zarb GA, Albrektsson T, editors. Tissue-integrated prostheses: osseointegration in clinical dentistry. Chicago: Quintessence Publishing Co; 1985. p. 99–116.

[32] Lautenschlager EP, Monaghan P. Titanium and titanium alloys as dental materials. Int Dent J 1993;43(3):245–53.

[33] De Rossi SS, Greenberg MS. Intraoral contact allergy: a literature review and case reports. J Am Dent Assoc 1998;129(10):1435–41.

[34] Hensten-Pettersen A. Skin and mucosal reactions associated with dental materials. Eur J Oral Sci 1998;106(2 Pt 2):707–12.

[35] Axéll T. Hypersensitivity of the oral mucosa: clinics and pathology. Acta Odontol Scand 2001;59(5):315–9.

[36] Gawkrodger DJ. Investigation of reactions to dental materials. Br J Dermatol 2005;153(3): 479–85.

[37] Albrektsson T. Bone tissue response. In: Brånemark P-I, Zarb GA, Albrektsson T, editors. Tissue-integrated prostheses: osseointegration in clinical dentistry. Chicago: Quintessence Publishing Co; 1985. p. 129–43.

[38] Tschemitschek H, Borchers L, Geurtsen W. Nonalloyed titanium as a bioinert metal – a review. Quintessense Int 2005;36(7/8):523–30.

[39] Wataha JC. Biocompatibility of dental materials. In: Craig RG, Powers JM, editors. Restorative dental materials. 11th edition. Philadelphia: Mosby; 2002. p. 125–62.

[40] Messer RLW, Lockwood PE, Wataha JC, et al. In vitro cytotoxicity of traditional versus contemporary dental ceramics. J Prosthet Dent 2003;90(5):452–8.

[41] Gosain AK. Plastic Surgery Educational Foundation DATA Committee. Bioactive glass for bone replacement in craniomaxillofacial reconstruction. Plast Reconstr Surg 2004;114(2): 590–3.

[42] Yuan H, de Bruijn JD, Zhang X, et al. Bone induction by porous glass ceramic made from bioglass (45S5). J Biomed Mater Res 2001;58(3):270–6.

[43] St. John KR, Zardiackas LD, Black RJ, et al. Response of bone to a synthetic bone graft material. Clin Mater 1993;12(1):49–55.

[44] St. John KR, Zardiackas LD, Terry RC, et al. Histological and electron microscopic analysis of tissue response to synthetic composite bone graft in the canine. J Appl Biomater 1995;6(2): 89–97.

[45] LeGeros RZ. Properties of osteoconductive biomaterials: calcium phosphates. Clin Orthop Relat Res 2002;395:81–98.

[46] Murray DW, Rushton N. Macrophages stimulate bone resorption when they phagocytose particles. J Bone Joint Surg [Br] 1990;72(6):988–92.

[47] Lassus J, Salo J, Jiranek WA, et al. Macrophage activation results in bone resorption. Clin Orthop Relat Res 1998;352:7–15.

[48] Horowitz SM, Rapuano BPO, Lane JM, et al. The interaction of the macrophage and the osteoblast in the pathophysiology of aseptic loosening of joint replacements. Calcif Tissue Int 1994;54(4):320–4.

[49] Archibeck MJ, Jacobs JJ, Roebuck KA, et al. The basic science of periprosthetic osteolysis. J Bone Joint Surg Am 2000;82A(10):1478–89.

[50] Spagnoli D, Kent JN. Multicenter evaluation of temporomandibular joint proplast-teflon disk implant. Oral Surg Oral Med Oral Pathol 1992;74(4):411–21.

[51] Kohn DH. Mechanical properties. In: Craig RG, Powers JM, editors. Restorative dental materials. 11th edition. Philadelphia: Mosby; 2002. p. 67–124.

[52] Anusavice KJ. Mechanical properties of dental materials. In: Anusavice KJ, editor. Phillips' science of dental materials. 11th edition. St. Louis (MO): Saunders; 2003. p. 73–102.

[53] Stanley HR. Toxicity testing of dental materials. Boca Raton (FL): CRC Press; 1985.

[54] Hanks CT, Wataha JC, Sun Z. In vitro models of biocompatibility: a review. Dent Mater 1996;12(3):186–93.

[55] Polyzois GL. In vitro evaluation of dental materials. Clin Mater 1994;16(1):21–60.

[56] Kinca J III. Pulpal studies: biocompatibility or effectiveness of marginal seal? Quintessense Int 1990;21(10):775–9.

[57] Recommended standard practices for biological evaluation of dental materials (ANSI/ADA Specification No. 41). Chicago: American Dental Association; 1979.

[58] Dentistry: preclinical evaluation of biocompatibility of medical devices used in dentistry. Test methods for dental materials (ISO 7405:1997(E)). Geneva (Switzerland): International Organization for Standardization;1997. (ISO Standards can be purchased from the American National Standards Institute [ANSI]). Available at: http://webstore.ansi.org/ansidocstore/default.asp.

[59] Biological evaluation of medical devices. I. Evaluation and testing (ANSI/AAMI/ISO 10993-1:2003). Geneva (Switzerland): International Organization for Standardization; 2003.

[60] Standard practice for selecting generic biological test methods for materials and devices (F748). In: ASTM standards on disc, vol. 13.01. West Conshohocken (PA): ASTM International; 2005.

[61] Dental impression materials: premarket notification. Rockville (MD): U.S. Food and Drug Administration; 1998.

[62] OTC denture cushions, pads, reliners, repair kits, and partially fabricated denture kits. Rockville (MD): U.S. Food and Drug Administration; 1998.

[63] Dental cements: premarket notification. Rockville (MD): U.S. Food and Drug Administration; 1998.

[64] Class II special controls guidance document: root-form endosseous dental implants and endosseous dental implant abutments. Rockville (MD): U.S. Food and Drug Administration; 2004.

[65] Class II special controls guidance document: dental base metal alloys. Rockville (MD): U.S. Food and Drug Administration; 2004.

[66] US Food and Drug Administration. Class II special controls guidance document: dental noble metal alloys. Rockville (MD): US Food and Drug Administration; 2004.

[67] Class II special controls guidance document: dental bone grafting material devices. Rockville (MD): U.S. Food and Drug Administration; 2005.

[68] Dental composite resin devices: premarket notification [510(k)] submissions. Rockville (MD): U.S. Food and Drug Administration; 2005.

[69] Special control guidance document on encapsulated amalgam, amalgam alloy, and dental mercury labeling: draft guidance for industry and FDA. Rockville (MD): U.S. Food and Drug Administration; 2002.

ELSEVIER
SAUNDERS

Dent Clin N Am 51 (2007) 761–765

THE DENTAL
CLINICS
OF NORTH AMERICA

Index

Note: Page numbers of article titles are in **boldface** type.

Moving?

Make sure your subscription moves with you!

To notify us of your new address, find your **Clinics Account Number** (located on your mailing label above your name), and contact customer service at:

E-mail: elspcs@elsevier.com

800-654-2452 (subscribers in the U.S. & Canada)
407-345-4000 (subscribers outside of the U.S. & Canada)

Fax number: 407-363-9661

Elsevier Periodicals Customer Service
6277 Sea Harbor Drive
Orlando, FL 32887-4800

*To ensure uninterrupted delivery of your subscription, please notify us at least 4 weeks in advance of move.